100 Plus Essential Oil And Organic Recipes Box Set

Over 300 Essential Oil Recipes For Beauty, Beauty Products, Bodyscrubs, Healing And Health (3 Books In 1)

SANDY COMFORT

Disclaimer

The information in this book is solely for informational purposes, not as a medical instruction to replace the advice of your physician or as a replacement for any treatment prescribed by your physician. The author and publisher do not take responsibility for any possible consequences from any treatment, procedure, exercise, dietary modification, action or application of medication which results from reading or following the information contained in this book.

If you are ill or suspect that you have a medical problem, we strongly encourage you to consult your medical, health, or other competent professional before adopting any of the suggestions in this book or drawing inferences from it.

This book and the author's opinions are solely for informational and educational purposes. The author specifically disclaims all responsibility for any liability, loss, or risk, personal or otherwise which is incurred as a consequence, directly or indirectly, of the use and application of any of the contents of this book.

DEDICATION

To everyone who made my dreams come true

TABLE OF CONTENTS

INTRODUCTION TO THE BOX SET

About Me

My name is Sandy Comfort. I believe in the use of organic and natural alternatives to everything we use. I believe in the healing powers of essential oils, the use of natural products and wellness treatments that are 100 percent natural, effective, affordable and tremendously beneficial.

I am also happy to know that my 100 plus essential oil books have garnered quite an audience in the last couple of years. So I believe the release of this box set will get to a far wider audience. Consider this book as a great reference book for everything essential oil as it covers virtually everything that essential oils can do for you.

About The Book

Here in this Box Set are my three best- selling 100 plus essential oil books.

Book 1: 100 Plus Homemade Essential Oil Beauty Recipes

Book 2: 100 Plus Simple Homemade Organic Body Scrub Recipes

Book 3: 100 Plus Essential Oil Healing Recipes

To make it easier to understand, there is only one table of contents. The recipes in the books are categorized and it is these categories that are highlighted in the table of contents.

Overall, this essential oil box set is informative, precise, simple, clear and enjoyable. You will be so glad you read it!

BOOK 1

100 Plus Homemade Essential Oil Beauty Recipes

Aromatherapy Preparations For Skin, Lip And Hair Care

(Body Scrubs, Perfumes, Lotions, Creams, Deodorants, Bath Salts, Soaps And More)

Introduction

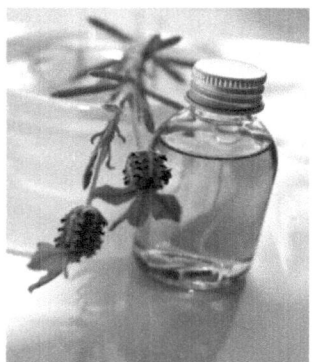

Nowadays, people are more health conscious than before. This is evident in the clamor for everything organic and natural. Whether it is our foods, clothing or beauty products, a large number of us now stay away from artificial additives having embraced the growing trend to go natural.

Using essential oil in our homemade beauty products such as perfumes, lotions, creams, cleansers, body scrubs and deodorants is one of the best ways to get the best out of our products. Extracted from plants, bark, roots, wood, flowers or seeds, essential oils are natural, highly concentrated oils with powerful antioxidant properties.

On my own part, I started experimenting with essential oils after being dissatisfied with the smells of store-bought products. In addition to the smells, these products contain chemicals that cause considerable damage to our skin. They are also very expensive. Then again, essential oils do a lot more than make you smell nice. They offer tremendous healing and purifying benefits.

Essential oils penetrate the skin easily. Within a few minutes, they are carried all through the blood and tissues. They increase the amount of oxygen that goes to the pineal and the pituitary glands. This ultimately increases the release of endorphins, antibodies and neurotransmitters which are healthy for the body.

Essential oil has multiple medicinal properties. Unlike most of our drugs that are meant for just one remedy, lavender essential oil for example, has analgesic, anti-inflammatory, sedative and antispasmodic properties. This means that it is suitable for pain, stress, sleeping and muscle cramps.

If kept in a cool dark place, essential oils usually last for up to 2 years. Only a few drops are required so they are very affordable.

Other benefits of essential oil:

- Prevent hair loss, improves hair quality
- Regenerate skin
- Support the immune system
- Sooth and promote healing of wounds, sunburn and scrapes
- Sooth digestive upsets
- sooth emotional issues
- Promote healthy thyroid and hormone function

Essential oil tips to remember:

- Do not use internally.
- Do not apply directly on your skin but dilute with carrier oil.
- Keep out children's reach.
- Avoid contact with eyes.
- Use only pure essential oils; stay away from synthetic fragrances.
- To avoid degradation and rancidity, store essential oils properly.

- Before experimenting with any oil, try to know its properties, precautions and dose.
- Do not use on children, pregnant women and the elderly

Use only essential oils that are safe for your skin.

HOMEMADE INVIGORATING BATH RECIPES

There is simply no reason to have a plain and unexciting bath time experience when there are several invigorating bath recipes to choose from. Containing essential oils, salts and other natural ingredients, these recipes are a healthy addition to your body. The inclusion of essential oils into your bath helps to hydrate and soften your skin as well as improve its tone and texture.

Bath salts contain anti-inflammatory properties and when combined with essential oils, you will have the opportunity of doubling the relief, rejuvenation and bliss that you'll enjoy. There are other bath recipes listed below such as bath bombs, bath cookies and bath teas. Take your pick and enjoy a healthy bath.

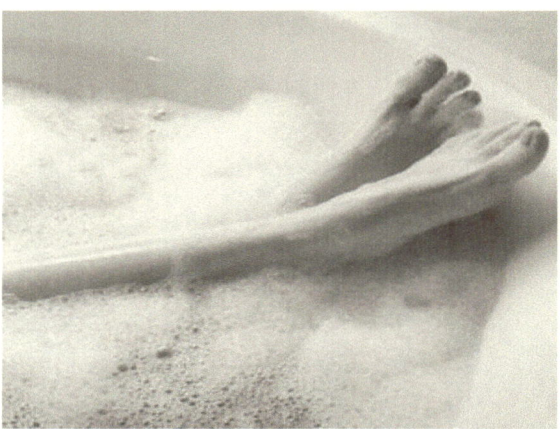

BATH OIL RECIPES

Simple Aromatherapy Bath Oil

<u>Ingredients:</u>

Essential oil of choice (15-30 drops)

Olive oil (1 1/2 oz)

Canola oil (1 oz)

Sesame oil (1 oz)

Almond oil (3 oz)

Wheat germ oil (1/2 oz)

<u>Directions:</u>

1. Fill a small- mouth jar with all the carrier oils.
2. Leave 1 /8 inch of space at the top.
3. Gradually add the essential oil.
4. use a tight lid to cap the jar and shake thoroughly
5. Use 2 teaspoons of oil per bath.

Use 2 teaspoons of oil per bath.

Blissful Oil Bath

Ingredients:

Sandalwood (10 drops)

Jasmine (5 drops)

Rose (5 drops)

Bergamot (5 drops)

Any of these base oils: Jojoba, Castor, Almond or simple Sunflower (4tbs)

Directions:

1. Pour base oil into a glass jar or bottle
2. Add essential oil. Cover and shake thoroughly.
3. Store in a dark place and leave for 2weeks to mature.
4. Once matured, add 1 tablespoon of the scented oil to the bath.
5. Swish to disburse.
6. Enjoy your blissful oil bath and remain happy.

Sensuous Oil Bath

Ingredients:

Jasmine (20 drops)

Orange (8 drops)

Any of these base oils: Jojoba, Castor, Almond or simple Sunflower (4tbs)

Directions:

Pour base oil into a glass jar or bottle.

Add essential oil. Cover and shake thoroughly.

Store in a dark place and leave for 2weeks to mature.

Once matured, add 1 tablespoon of the scented oil to the bath.

Swish to disburse.

Enjoy your sensual oil bath.

Revitalizing Oil Bath

Ingredients:

Geranium (12 drops)

Sandalwood (6 drops)

Lemon (6 drops)

Clary Sage (2 drops)

Any of these base oils: Jojoba, Castor, Almond or simple Sunflower (4tbs)

Directions

Pour base oil into a glass jar or bottle

Add essential oil. Cover and shake thoroughly.

Store in a dark place and leave for 2weeks to mature.

Once matured, add 1 tablespoon of the scented oil to the bath

Swish to disburse

Enjoy your revitalizing oil bath to relive stress and depression.

Relaxing Oil

Ingredients:

Sandalwood (12 drops)

Orange (8 drops)

Rose (4 drops)

Pine (2 drops)

Lemon (2 drops)

Any of these base oils: Jojoba, Castor, Almond or simple Sunflower (4tbs)

Directions

Pour base oil into a glass jar or bottle

Add essential oil. Cover and shake thoroughly.

Store in a dark place and leave for 2weeks to mature.

Once matured, add 1 tablespoon of the scented oil to the bath

Swish to disburse

Enjoy your relaxing oil bath to relive stress and depression

Shampoo Bath Oil

Ingredients:

Essential oil of choice (10 drops)

Mild baby shampoo (4 tbsp)

Almond or Sunflower Oil (125ml)

Note:

Baby shampoo is an effective carrier that helps to quickly and evenly disburse your oils.

Direction:

Pour base oil into a glass jar.

Add the shampoo and shake well

Add essential oil, shake well

Leave for 2 weeks to mature but keep way from daylight.

Once matured, add 2 tablespoons per bath and swish to disperse

Enjoy your bath.

Alcohol Bath Oil

Ingredients:

Castor Oil (100ml)

Vodka or brandy (4 tbsp)

Essential oils of choice (10 drops)

Note:

Spirits help in the quick and even distribution of the oil.

Direction

Pour the castor oil into a glass jar.

Add the spirit and shake well

Add essential oil, shake well

Leave for 2 weeks to mature but keep way from daylight.

Once matured, add 2 tablespoons per bath and swish to disperse

Enjoy your bath.

Here Are My 10 Best Singular Bath Oil Recipes:

Treatment	Essential oil	Quantity
Depression	Bergamot oil	5 drops
Stress or fatigue	Jasmine	8 drops
Soothing and relaxing	Lavender	10 drops
Insomnia or itchy skin	Chamomile	7 drops
Sensual and mellowing a great aphrodisiac	Sandalwood	8 drops
Happiness and romantic pleasure	Rose	10 drops
Relaxing, uplifting and energizing	Geranium	10 drops
hypnotic with antidepressant properties	Neroli	7 drops

energizing and invigorating	Patchouli	5 drops
sedative and mood sweetening	Frankincense	8 drops

BATH SALT RECIPES

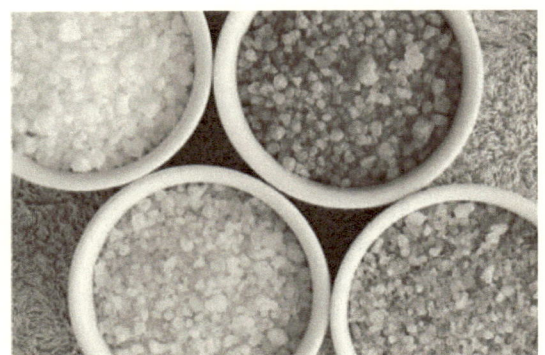

Lemon Bath Salt Recipe

Ingredients:

Fine grain Sea Salt (1 cup)

Epsom Salt (1 cup)

Dendritic salt (ideal for making scented bath salts, 3 tbsp)

Lemon essential oil (1/2 tsp)

Vanilla Extract (1/2 tsp)

Yellow 5 liquid dye (5 drops)

Directions:

Pour the fine grain Sea Salt and the Epsom Salt into a large stainless steel mixing bowl and then set aside.

In a separate but smaller mixing bowl, pour in the dendritic salt and add the vanilla extract and the lemon essential oil.

Mix very thoroughly and then add this mixture to the salts in the large stainless steel mixing bowl.

Mix thoroughly. Add yellow dye to the salt mixture and continue to mix well until the color is even throughout

Either use immediately or package well.

Margarita Bath Salt Recipe

Ingredients:

Epsom salts (1 cup)

Green food coloring (4-5 drops)

Lime essential oil (10 drops)

Directions:

Combine all the ingredients: Epsom salts, essential oil and coloring and mix well.

Pour into in a small glass jar and seal.

Leave it to set for several days.

Store in plastic bags or decorative jars.

Add bath salts into hot running or warm bath water.

Soak liberally.

Seaside Bath Salt Soak

Ingredients:

Epsom Salt (210 grams)

Kelp Powder (9 grams)

Powdered Grapefruit Peel (6 grams)

Spirulina Powder (3 grams)

Olive Oil (40 grams)

Rosemary Essential Oil (60 drops)

Juniper Essential Oil (30 drops)

Eucalyptus Essential Oil (20 drops)

Notes:

Grapefruit Peel powder, Kelp powder and Spirulina powder improves skin tone and promotes the synthesis of new collagen.

Epsom salt is ideal for soothing, relaxing and relieving sore muscles.

You may also use Sea Salt just add a few scoops of it to warm running bath water.

Be careful because this product contains oil and oil is slippery.

Directions:

Mix all the ingredients in a small bowl.

Transfer to a glass jar and use within 60 days.

This recipe may cause the bath surface to become very slippery so be careful while using it.

Aromatherapy Bath Salts Recipe

Ingredients:

Epsom salts (2 1/2 cups)

Baking Soda (1 cup)

Citric Acid (1/2 cup)

Sweet Almond Oil (2 1/2 tsp)

Ginger, peppermint and eucalyptus essential Oils (about 60 drops)

Directions

In a mixing bowl, combine all the dry ingredients until the entire clumps are broken.

Mix your essential oils and set aside. Add the sweet almond oil to your essential oils recipe.

Mix them all together and blend thoroughly.

Package in a plastic bag.

Oatmeal, Milk And Honey Salt Bath

Ingredients:

Powdered full cream/whole milk (4 cups)

Ground oats (1 cup)

Ground plain, raw almonds (1 cup)

Baking soda (1/2 cup)

Sea salt (1 cup)

Honey (2 cups)

Vanilla Essential oil (4 drops)

Notes:

Milk : Contains lactic acid which helps in breaking down and dissolving the proteins that hold together the dead skin cells. These dead skin cells must be removed in order for fresh new ones to resurface leading to a total youthful looking skin.

Honey : can absorb and retain moisture and this is why it is an essential ingredient in this recipe. It has natural antibacterial antifungal and antioxidant properties as well and this facilitates healing of different skin problems.

Oatmeal as well as baking soda is a wonderful exfoliant helps to soothe and heal rashes, sunburn and skin irritations. Grind oatmeal so that it will easily blend with the bath water and milk. It also draws toxin.

Directions:

Combine the sea salt, almond, oats, bathing soda and milk and then mix thoroughly.

Dissolve 4 cups of this powdered mixture in warm bath water (alternatively, you may pour the mix mixture into a cheesecloth bag, a clean sock or coffee filter, tie it securely with a string and then soak in the bath water).

Add the honey and vanilla essential oil in the bath water and mix it thoroughly so it completely dissolves.

Soak your body in the bath for about 15 minutes.

Rinse out the milk body under a warm shower.

Gently dry your skin with a clean towel.

Ocean Bath Salts

Ingredients:

Epsom salt (1 cup)

Glycerin (2 tbsp)

Baking soda (1 cup)

Vanilla (4 drops)

Blue food coloring (4 drops)

Essential oil (3 drops)

Directions:

Combine dry ingredients and mix well.

Add scents and color one at a time.

Continue to stir until thoroughly mixed.

Break up any clumps.

Keep on mixing until a semi fine powder is formed.

Add glycerin and mix well.

OTHER BATH RECIPES

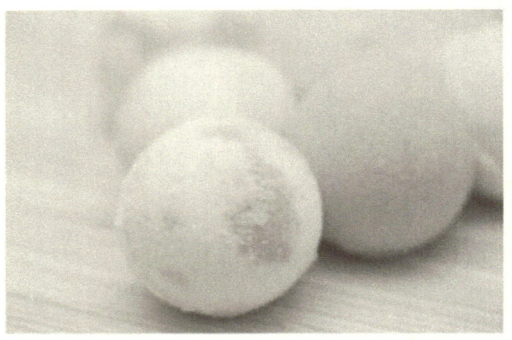

Plain Milk Bath

Ingredients:

Non-fat powdered milk (2 cups)

Cornstarch (1 cup)

Essential oil (5 drops)

Directions:

Mix ingredients well.

Add 1/2 cup to hot bath and enjoy a refreshing bath.

Meadow Milk Bath

Ingredients:

Finely sifted Powdered Milk (4 oz)

Citric Acid (2 oz)

Corn starch (2 oz)

Grapefruit Seed Oil (30 drops)

Jasmine essential oil (60 drops)

Directions

Blend the corn starch and powdered milk and then sift.

Mix the grapefruit seed oil and Jasmine in Citric Acid.

Make sure the oils are well blended in the Citric Acid.

Add the Citric Acid blend to the milk/corn starch blend.

Use 3 tablespoons to each bath.

Relaxing Bath Tea

Ingredients:

Lavender flowers (4 oz.)

Chamomile flowers (4 oz.)

Calendula petals (2 oz)

Bulgarian Lavender EO (20 drops)

Directions

Combine ingredients and package.

Scented Bath Bombs

Ingredients:

Baking soda (1 1/2 cups)

Citric acid 1/2 cup

Essential oil of choice (8 drops)

Sweet almond oil (1/2 tsp)

Food coloring of choice (2 drops)

Directions

Combine all the ingredients.

Press into mould or muffin tin of choice.

Release from mould.

Wrap in plastic wraps and tie with a ribbon.

Silky Body Wash

Ingredients:

Shea butter (1 tbsp)

Aloe Vera gel (1/4 cup)

Guar gum (3/4 tsp)

Castile Soap (3/4 cup)

Essential oils of choice (25 drops)

Directions:

Melt the Shea butter over low heat.

Add aloe Vera gel to the Shea butter and warm together.

Add gum and use a whisk to stir thoroughly.

Add the soap base.

Mix thoroughly in a blender to get the gum fully distributed.

After blending, your wash will appear foamy but will settle in a couple of hours.

Pour some in your bath or use in the shower.

Lavender & Chamomile Bath Melts

Ingredients:

Organic Shea butter (50g)

Organic cocoa butter (50g)

Lavender essential oil (2 drops)

Dried lavender flowers (1 tsp)

Organic chamomile tea (1 tsp)

Directions:

Thinly grate the cocoa butter and pour in a glass bowl. Add the Shea butter as well.

Place your glass bowl on a pan of hot water, stir until it melts then remove from heat.

Sprinkle organic chamomile tea into the mix. Add the dried lavender and stir thoroughly.

Pour the molten mix carefully into silicone moulds (ice cube trays can also be used).

Add the lavender essential oil to the moulds.

Refrigerate your melts for an hour so its hardens

Pop the melts from their mould and store in a fine glass jar.

How To Use:

Pop a bath melt in a warm bath and then wait till it dissolves.

The cocoa butter may make your bath a little slippery so you've got to be careful.

However, you can put your bath melt in a muslin cloth bag if you do not want the chamomile and lavender flowers to cover your bath.

HOMEMADE SOAP RECIPES

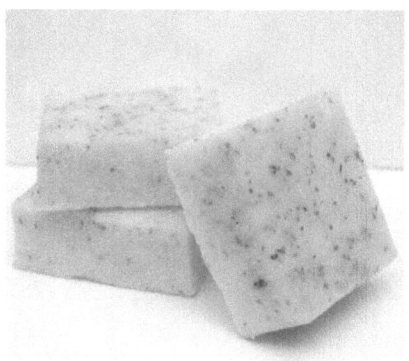

Homemade Lemon Soap

Ingredients:

Goat's milk soap base (13 cubes)

Lemon essential oil

Lemon zest of 3-4 lemons (optional)

Directions:

Cut the soap into cubes.

Melt soap for about 2 minutes using a large pyrex measuring cup.

As soon as soap cubes turn liquid, add the lemon zest and some drops of the lemon essential oil and stir well.

Pour into soap molds. Leave for one hour to harden.

Press mold to release soap.

Seaweed Soap

Ingredients:

Clear soap base (32 ounces)

Dried seaweed (6-8 pieces)

Extra virgin olive oil (1 teaspoon)

Lemon essential oil (1.5 teaspoons)

Lavender essential oil (1 teaspoon)

Dash of green mica

Mold: 3 part Ziploc, divided rectangle mold

Directions:

Place seaweed pieces into mold.

Slice the soap base into tiny cubes.

Add the essential oils, colorant and olive oil just before the soap is completely melted, stir well.

Slowly pour into the molds.

Leave soap in freezer or fridge to harden. It may remain in at room temperature, however.

Remove from molds.

Once the soap is at room temperature, cut and wrap.

Hand Wash Liquid Soap

Ingredients:

Liquid Soap (1 cup)

Water (1 cup)

Essential oils of choice (8 drops)

Directions:

Mix ingredients together

Pour into a bottle

Shake thoroughly

Antibacterial & Antiviral Hand Wash Soap

Ingredients:

Liquid Soap (1 cup)

Water (1 cup)

Essential oils of choice (8 drops)

Tea Tree oil (3 drops)

Lavender oil (5 drops)

Directions:

Mix ingredients together

Pour into a bottle

Shake thoroughly.

Sweet Honey Soap

Ingredients:

Castile soap (1 lb)

Honey (1/4 lb)

Glycerin (1/4 lb)

Sandalwood essential oil (5drops)

Fine oatmeal (2 tbsp)

Directions:

Grate the soap.

Put some water in the pot

Add the honey, glycerin, the oatmeal and essential oil.

Mix well until soap is dissolved.

Boil for 3 minutes, pour into soap moulds or a deep wet container.

Cut into pieces when it is quite cold.

Leave out until it's dry before storing.

Lavender Soap

Ingredients:

Unscented soap (1)

Dried lavender (1)

Lavender essential oil (3 drops)

Directions:

Grate a bar unscented soap and place inside some water in a bowl.

Place the bowl in a pan of hot water. stir thoroughly until smooth

Add the dried lavender flowers to the soap.

Remove the bowl from pan

Add lavender essential oil

Pour into molds.

Simple Soap Recipe

Ingredients:

Castile Soap Flakes and or/Glycerin Soap (1 lb)

Fennel essential oil (8 drops)

Grapefruit essential oil (14 drops)

Lemon essential oil (8 drops)

Purified Water (1 cup)

Herbal Tea or Hydrosol (1/2 cup)

Directions:

Melt the glycerin in double boiler hydrosol or herbal infusion.

Leave it to cool for a while.

Add essential oil and stir thoroughly.

Pour into moulds

Leave to harden and cut into bars.

Use a knife to smooth rough spots.

Herbal Soap

Ingredients:

Block olive or veg. soap (1g)

Loosely chopped herbs (25 g)

Thyme or rosemary essential oil (3 drops)

Finely ground oatmeal (1 tbsp)

Directions:

Grate the soap into a bowl and add the remaining ingredients.

Heat gently till it melts.

Mix well.

Pour soup into each section of an egg box that has been lined with waxed paper.

Basic Lotion Bars

Ingredients:

Beeswax (2 oz)

Almond oil (1 oz)

Cocoa butter (1 oz)

Essential oil (3drops)

Directions:

Melt cocoa butter and beeswax and on the stove in a clean pot.

Once it melts, remove from heat and then add the almond oil.

 Mix in the essential oil drop by drop until it's attains the desired scent.

Pour the mixture into a mould.

Leave it to it set fully before using.

HAIR CARE RECIPES

Several hair growth care and treatments depend on essential oils. Essential oils are versatile and can work wonders on any type of hair and scalp. Some of them work directly on the hair by helping to strengthen and repair it. Others help to improve the condition of the scalp alone.

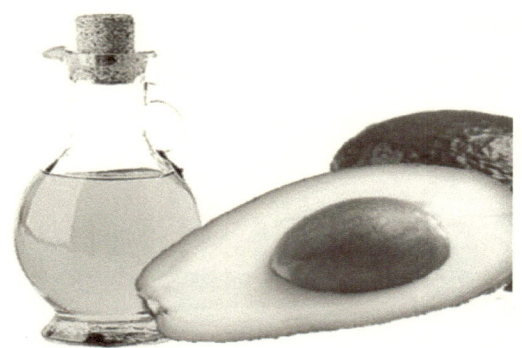

Essential Oils For Split Ends

<u>Ingredients:</u>

Sandalwood essential oil (10 drops)

Rosemary essential oil (10 drops)

<u>Directions:</u>

Combine ingredients

Use your fingers to rub them in.

Avocado Hair Moisturizing Recipe

Ingredients:

Half avocado

Peppermint essential oil (few drops)

Oil (1-2 tbsp, optional)

Egg yolk (1-2 tbsp, optional)

Directions:

Mash the avocado up.

Add the essential oil

Shampoo your hair, squeeze the water out and apply mask.

Allow to sit for 15minutes. Rinse off.

Hair will come out super soft and smell real nice.

Homemade Hair Softener/ Growth Recipe

Ingredients:

Thyme essential oil (2 drops)

Cedar essential oil (2 drops)

Rosemary essential oil (3 drops)

Grapeseed (1 ounce)

Jojoba (1 tbsp)

Directions:

Mix all the ingredients in a bowl.

Pour into a tight bottle for easy storage.

Every night, massage the mixture into your scalp.

Rinse in cool water and shampoo the next morning.

For oily hair, 3 times in a week is fine.

This recipe promotes hair growth and softens hair.

Sweet-Smelling Herbal Shampoo

Ingredients:

Unscented shampoo (2 ounces)

Chamomile essential oil (12 drops)

Lavender essential oil (12 drops)

Directions:

Mix all the ingredients

Shake well before use.

Warm Oil Recipe For Dry Hair

Ingredients:

Aloe Vera gel (2 ounces)

Castor oil (2 ounces)

Rose geranium cedar essential oil (6 drops)

Rosemary essential oil (8 drops)

Ginger essential oil (2 drops)

Directions:

Combine all the ingredients

Warm the mixture and apply to scalp and hair in sections

Use a towel to cover the head and leave it on for an hour and

Wash off.

After Shampooing Rinse: For Dry Hair

Ingredients:

Comfrey oil (2 tsp)

Marshmallow oil (2 tsp)

Parsley essential oil (2 drops)

Sage essential oil (2 drops)

Water (4 cups)

Vinegar (2cups)

Directions:

Combine all the ingredients.

Rinse your hair with this mixture after shampooing.

Keep it away from your eyes.

The Rinse can be reused once or twice.

Henna Protein Treatment

Ingredients:

Henna (3 ounces)

Honey (2 tbsp)

Lavender essential oil (24 drops)

Warm water (2 cups)

Olive oil (1 tsp)

Egg (1)

Directions:

Mix all the ingredients

Add this mixture to henna, remove any lumps.

Wet the hair and apply from roots to ends.

Keep the heat in by covering for 1 or 2 hours with a plastic bag and towel.

The henna breaks down and the color becomes darker when you do this but ensure that the henna doesn't dry out.

Rinse several times with warm water, and then apply shampoo and conditioner to it.

Make sure you use gloves and wear an apron to avoid staining your skin.

Deep Endings Essential Oil Treatment

The ends of your hair will be nourished by this revitalizing oil treatment. Its usefulness is more pronounced in the winter when hair tends to rub up against heavy fabrics, including wools.

Ingredients:

Sweet almond, olive or peanut oil (1-3 tsp)

Pure lavender essential oil (2-4 drops)

Note:

The quantity of the peanut, olive or sweet almond oil depends on how long or thick your hair is

Directions:

Combine the oils and apply it to the end of your hair.

Using a clear plastic wrap, wrap the hair and leave for about 30 minutes.

Rinse with Lemon Aid.

Lavender Mist

Ingredients:

Water (½ gallon)

Lavender essential oil (5 drops)

Directions:

Pour the half gallon of water in a large pot.

Cover, boil and let it simmer for 1 hour so as to remove impurities.

(Distilled water can also be used).

Remove from heat and then add the lavender oil

Stir thoroughly, leave to cool

Pour into spritz bottles

Lavender helps to cleanse and revive your hair.

Homemade Hair Conditioner Oil

Ingredients:

Jojoba oil (1 tablespoon)

Rosemary essential oil (3 drops)

Directions:

Mix the essential oil (Rosemary) and jojoba in a small bow

Wet your hair with warm water, apply the mixture and leave it to sit on your hair for 30 minutes.

Wash your hair afterwards.

Scaly Scalp And Dandruff Blend Recipe

Ingredients:

Atlas cedar- wood (2 drops)

Rosemary (2 drops)

Lavender (2 drops)

Tea tree oil (2 drops)

Jojoba (1/2 ounce)

Directions

Mix all ingredients together.

Apply on scalp

Scented Hair Gel

Ingredients:

Water (1 cup)

Flax seed (2 tbsp)

Essential oil (2 drops)

Directions:

In a small saucepan, mix water and seed.

Bring to boil and then remove from heat.

Allow to set for 30minutes and then strain.

Once cooled, add essential oil

Pour into to a wide-mouthed container with lid.

Quality Hair Treatment

This recipe is ideal for a thicker, smoother and nice- smelling hair.

Ingredients:

Honey (2 spoons)

Olive oil (2 spoons)

Eggs (2)

Rose EO (10 drops)

Lavender EO (5 drops)

Directions:

Combine all ingredients

Apply all over the hair.

Leave for an hour

Wash away.

LIP BALM RECIPES
<u>Note:</u>

All recipes should be thrown away once it changes odor, texture or color.

Vitamin E Capsule is used as a preservative.

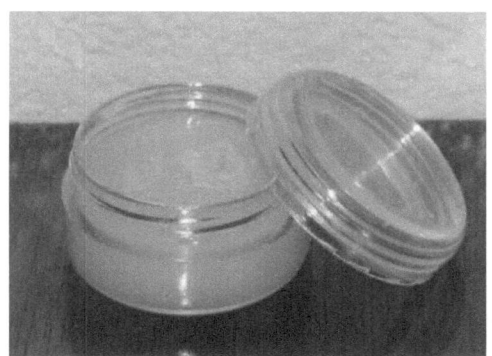

Honey Cocoa Lip Balm

<u>Ingredients:</u>

Olive oil (2 tsp)

Cocoa butter (½ tsp)

Honey (½ tsp)

Beeswax (½ tsp)

Orange essential oil (3 drops)

Vitamin E capsule (1)

Direction:

Place the cocoa butter, oil and beeswax into a glass pan.

Use a hotplate to melt over low heat.

Stir until thoroughly melted. Remove from heat

Add the honey and essential oil into it.

Squeeze the vitamin E capsule into the mixture and stir.

Pour the mixture into fine containers.

Honey Balm

Ingredients

Almond Oil (3 oz)

Beeswax or Beeswax Pellets (½ oz.)

Honey (2 Teaspoons)

Essential Oil (1-4 Drops)

Vitamin E capsule (1)

Directions:

Mix the beeswax and almond oil together in a bowl.

Place bowl in a pan of water and heat on a stovetop.

Heat until mixture is fully melted, stirring continuously to completely melt the wax.

Remove from heat and add the honey and essential oil in it.

Open the vitamin E capsule, squeeze the contents into it.

Stir the mixture one more time

Allow it to completely cool

Once cool, pour into small plastic containers.

Peppermint Flavored Lip Balm

Ingredients:

Petroleum jelly (2 tbsp)

Beeswax (1 tsp)

Peppermint essential oil (10-14 drops)

Directions:

Melt the petroleum jelly in a small pot.

Add in the beeswax.

Remove from the heat once melted.

Now add the peppermint essential oil.

Pour into a lip pot

Leave to cool.

Tangerine Lip Gloss

Ingredients:

Beeswax (2 tsp)

Honey (1 tsp)

Sweet almond, jojoba or castor oil (7 tsp)

Tangerine essential oil (5 drops)

Directions:

Melt the beeswax and oil until completely melted.

Remove from heat and then add the honey.

Whisk it all up.

When the mixture is almost cool, add the essential oil and mix it up again.

Pour into a container.

Lemon Lip Gloss

Ingredients:

Beeswax (2 tsp)

Honey (1 tsp)

Sweet almond, jojoba or castor oil (7 tsp)

Lemon essential oil (5 drops)

Directions:

Melt the beeswax and oil until completely melted.

Remove from heat and then add the honey.

Whisk it all up.

When the mixture is almost cool, add the essential oil and mix it up again.

Pour into a container.

To make it harder, add more beeswax

Hemp Oil Lip Balm

Ingredients:

Coconut oil (3 tbsp)

Castor oil

Sunflower oil (1 tbsp)

Hemp seed oil (1 tbsp)

Beeswax (1 tbsp)

Honey (1 tbsp)

Peppermint essential oil (few drops)

Directions:

Melt the coconut oil and wax together.

Add the honey and heat for some time.

Stir continuously and add the sunflower and castor oil.

As the mixture thickens, add the peppermint essential oil and the hempseed oil.

Stir until it thickens.

Rosey-Coco Lip Balm Recipe

Ingredients:

Coconut oil (2 Tbsp)

Grated cocoa butter (1 Tbsp)

Dried rosebuds (or any dried flower etc, 1 Tbsp)

Vitamin E oil (1/4 tsp)

Rose, vanilla or lavender essential oil (3 drops)

Directions:

Place the coconut oil in a stainless steel bowl and melt over very low heat.

Once melted, add the roses (or any dried flowers of your choice) and stir thoroughly.

Place on very low heat again for an hour.

Use a cheesecloth or fine-mesh sieve to sieve the oil into a bowl

Clean your original heating bowl and pour the oil back in. Return to heat.

Add the cocoa butter and stir until well melted. Remove from heat.

Add essential oil and vitamin E oil and stir well.

Transfer to a container and leave it for 3 hours to set.

Note:

Remember this is mostly coconut oil so do not put this recipe in a lip balm tube. Do not keep in your pocket, either. Coconut oil liquefies quickly when it is in contact with only a small amount of heat. Even keeping it in a warm place like your body will make it leak all over.

Minty Choc Lip Balm Recipe

Ingredients:

Beeswax pearls or grated beeswax (1 Tbsp)

Coconut oil (1/8 cup)

Shear butter (1/2 Tbsp)

Cocoa butter (1/2 Tbsp)

Honey (1/2 tsp)

Cocoa powder (1 tsp)

Vitamin E oil (1/8 tsp)

Peppermint essential oil (3 drops)

Directions:

In a small pot, place the cocoa and Shea butters and add the coconut oil.

Heat over extremely low heat for 20 minutes. Stir occasionally. (Do not let the mixture go beyond 175 degrees else the Shea butter will become a little gritty.)

Add in the beeswax and stir.

When the beeswax is completely melted, remove from heat.

Add the honey, cocoa powder, essential oil, and vitamin E, whisking thoroughly the whole time.

Once everything is incorporated, transfer to a lip balm tin and leave for 3hours to set.

Sweet Lavender Lip Balm Recipe

Ingredients:

Beeswax pearls or grated beeswax (1 tbsp)

Honey (1 tsp)

Cocoa powder (1 tsp, optional)

Jojoba, olive or almond oil (4 tbsp)

Vitamin E oil (1/4 tsp)

Lavender essential oil (7 drops)

Colored, natural lipstick to give it a hint of color (optional, 1 tsp)

Directions:

Warm the honey, oils and beeswax on very low heat in a small bowl.

Stir until the beeswax is totally melted. Remove from heat.

Quickly whisk in the colored lipstick, cocoa powder, essential oil and vitamin E.

Place the bowl into a pan of ice water and keep on whisking as you add the honey.

Once the honey is fully incorporated, transfer the balm quickly into your lip balm container

Leave to set for 3 hours.

Note

Mineral eye shadow tubs make great lip balm containers so do not throw yours away after use. It's fun to be creative. Match and mix colors until you find the one you love.

Cold Sores Treatment Lip Balm

Ingredients:

Emu Oil (1 oz)

Almond Oil (1 oz)

Avocado Oil (1 oz)

Beeswax Pellets or Shaved Beeswax (1 /2 oz.)

Aloe Vera Gel (1/4 oz.)

Lavender Essential Oil (6 Drops)

Tea Tree Essential Oil (2 Drops)

Lime Essential Oil (3 Drops)

Directions:

Mix the beeswax, emu, almond and avocado oil together in a bowl.

Heat the bowl in a pan of water on a stove

Stir the mixture repeatedly until the beeswax is melted.

Add the aloe Vera gel.

Remove from heat, add the essential oils and stir.

Stir once more and leave to completely cool.

Transfer into small plastic tins when cool

Sweet Sugar Lip Balm Recipe

Ingredients:

Sweet almond oil (20 ml)

Grated beeswax or beeswax pellets (½ tsp)

Cocoa butter (½ tsp)

Icing sugar (1 tsp)

Vitamin E (1 capsule)

Peppermint, sweet orange or rose essential oil (5 drops)

Directions:

Melt cocoa butter, beeswax and oil in a double boiler

Add the icing sugar and stir so it dissolves.

Remove from heat and then add the vitamin E by puncturing the capsule and pouring oil in.

Add the essential oils, stir again and pour into a lip balm container.

Luscious Lip Balm Recipe

<u>Ingredients:</u>

Filtered, raw beeswax1 tbsp (0.5 oz)

Unscented coconut oil (4 tbsp)

Bergamot essential oil (10 drops)

<u>Directions:</u>

Add beeswax and coconut oil to a glass measuring cup.

Microwave every 30 second until beeswax is melted.

Remove the mixture from the microwave and set aside

Add the essential oil to the mixture, stirring carefully.

Pour slowly into your lip balm tins.

Leave at room temperature to cool and set.

HOMEMADE DEODORANTS AND POWDERS

A lot of people react very strongly to store-bought deodorant. Homemade deodorants are a healthy alternative and they cost much less as well.

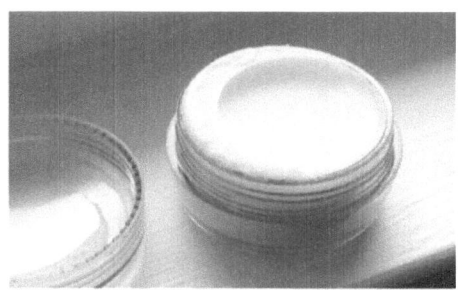

Scented Orange Deodorant Powder

Ingredients:

Baking soda (3 tsps)

Arrowroot powder (2tbs)

Cornflour (2tbs)

Sweet orange essential oil (10 drops)

Neroli essential oil (10 drops)

Directions:

Mix all the dry ingredients in bowl.

Add the essential oils, mix well.

Store in an airtight container.

Simple Deodorant Powder

Ingredients:

Coconut Oil (3tbsp)

Baking Soda (3tbsp)

Shea Butter (2tbsp)

Arrowroot (2tbsp)

Essential Oils (5drops)

Directions:

Melt coconut oil and Shea butter in a double boiler over low heat until barely melted. Remove from heat. Add arrowroot and baking soda. Mix well. Add essential oils and pour into a glass container for storage

Fairy Dusting Powder

Ingredients:

Rice Flour (1/2 cup)

Cornstarch (1/2 cup)

Finely ground Rose petals (2 tsp)

Mica, very fine glitter (1/2 tsp)

Essential Oil (3 drops)

Directions:

Mix all the dry ingredients together. Add essential oil and mix thoroughly. Put in an airtight container.

Pineapple Deodorant Powder

Ingredients

Coconut oil (1 tbsp)

Baking soda (1 cup)

Powdered coconut milk (1/2 cups)

Pineapple essential oil (1 tbsp)

Directions

Melt coconut oil and Set aside. Mix coconut powder and baking soda in a tight-lid container.

Add essential oil and the melted coconut oil.

Use a powder brush or puff to apply the deodorant.

Face Powder Foundation

Ingredients

Cornstarch or arrowroot powder (2 tbsp)

Cinnamon, nutmeg or cocoa powder (1½ tsp, add more as necessary for tinting)

Essential oil (5 drops)

Directions

Mix all the ingredients in a bowl. Stir until well mixed.

Add tint (cocoa powder, cinnamon or nutmeg) until you attain your desired color.

Keep adding any of these tints until you get a similar tone for your skin.

Fine Thyme Deodorant Powder

Ingredients:

Arrowroot (1 1/2 c)

Baking soda/ bicarbonate of soda (1 cup)

Finely powdered thyme (1/4 c)

Calcium bentonite clay (1/4 c)

Zeolite powder (1 tbsp)

Rosemary essential oil (100 drops)

Thyme essential oil (50 drops)

Directions

Combine all the ingredients except the essential oils in a large bowl.

Blend in a food processor for 20 seconds or whisk by hand.

Slowly add the essential oils to 7 tablespoons of the powder mix. Use a mortar and pestle.

Add oil mixture to the rest of the powder and whirl for 20 seconds in a food processor.

Let the mixture sit for 3 days so that the oils can permeate the powder.

Place in a small jar.

Homemade Deodorant For Men

Ingredients:

Vodka (50 ml)

Pure witch hazel (50 ml)

Sandalwood (15 drops)

Black pepper (5 drop)

Cypress (10 drops)

Frankincense (5 drops)

Tea tree (5 drops)

Directions:

Add the oils into your glass bottle

Add the vodka and witch hazel.

Close firmly with the sprayer and cap.

Shake thoroughly before each use so as to redistribute the oils.

Homemade Probiotic Deodorant

Ingredients:

Cocoa butter (1 tbsp)

Coconut oil (1 tbsp)

Shea butter (1 tbsp)

Beeswax (1 tbsp)

Arrowroot powder (2 1/2 tbsp)

Baking soda (1 tbsp)

Vitamin E oil (1/4 tsp)

Essential oils of choice (15 drops)

Powdered probiotics (2 capsules)

Directions

Melt Shea butter, coconut oil, cocoa butter and beeswax over very low heat.

Remove pot from heat. Add baking soda and arrowroot powder into it

Whisk until all powders are dissolved and mixed.

Add essential oils and vitamin E oil. Allow mixture to cool.

Once it is cooled, open the capsules of probiotics and add powder to the mixture.

Stir quickly with spatula to combine. Add mixture to used but clean deodorant container.

Place in refrigerator to cool and harden. Store afterwards.

Lasts for for3-4 months.

Lemony Deodorant Recipe

Ingredients:

Extra virgin coconut oil (1-1/3 cups)

Beeswax shavings (1-1/2 tablespoons)

Baking soda (1/4 cup)

Arrowroot powder (3/4 cup)

Clay (2 tbsp)

Tea tree essential oil (25 drops)

Lemongrass essential oil (5 drops)

Directions:

Melt beeswax and coconut oil over low heat until barely melted.

Remove from heat and then add the remaining ingredients apart from essential oils.

Leave to cool while stirring continuously until it hardens.

Refrigerate to speed this up. Check and stir frequently.

Add essential oils and thoroughly combine.

Pour into empty deodorant containers.

Leave in a cool location or refrigerate to harden.

For each arm, use about 1/8 teaspoon.

Simply Fresh Deodorant Powder

Ingredients:

Coconut oil (6 tbsp)

Baking soda (4 tbsp)

Arrowroot or cornstarch (4 T)

Essential oils (5 drops)

Directions:

In a medium sized bowl, mix arrowroot and baking soda together.

Use a fork to mash in coconut oil until well mixed.

Add essential oil

Store in a used deodorant container for easy use.

Rich Deodorant Spray

Ingredients:

Vodka (50 ml)

Pure witch hazel (50 ml)

Ylang ylang (10 drops)

Geranium (10 drops)

Bergamot (10 drops)

Sandalwood (10 drops)

Directions:

Add the oils into your glass bottle. Add the vodka and witch hazel. Close firmly with the sprayer and cap. Shake thoroughly before each use so as to redistribute the oils.

Herbal Deodorant Powder

Ingredients:

Powdered sandalwood (2 parts)

Powdered white oak bark (1 part)

Powdered lovage root (1 part)

Directions:

Pulverize herbs in a food processor or blender until they are in powdered form.

Transfer powder into an iron skillet. Pan-roast gently. Pour powdered herbs into a muslin draw-string bags. Pat bags on your feet or under your arms.

Sage Deodorizing Powder For Foot

Ingredients:

Baking powder (1 tbsp)

Sage essential oil (2 drops)

Directions:

Mix oil and baking powder in a plastic bag.

Shake thoroughly. Set aside to dry.

Break up any formed clumps.

Use powder to regularly dust feet

Leave a teaspoon in the shoes overnight.

BODY SCRUB RECIPES

Body scrubs are just great! They work by removing old layers of dead skin, leaving you with a fresh, glowing and healthy skin. There are two major types: salt and sugar. Salt will sting if you have scratches, or rashes. Sugar scrubs are gentler on the skin and also non-stinging so they are ideal for sensitive or irritated skin.

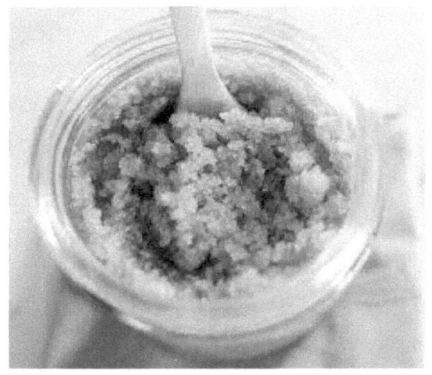

Sweet Sugar Scrub Recipe

Ingredients:

Sugar (3/4 cup)

Honey (1/4 cup)

Vegetable glycerin (1/8 cup)

Olive oil (1/8 cup)

Castile soap (or 1/4 liquid)

Your favorite essential oil (25 drops)

Directions:

Mix all the ingredients together in a bowl. Apply generously after showering, concentrating on areas like the elbows and knees. Rinse off. Apply any moisturizing body lotion.

Peppermint Sugar Scrub

Ingredients:

White granulated sugar (2 cups)

Almond oil (/4 cup)

Peppermint essential oil (5drops)

Raspberry/pomegranate juice (few drops)

Directions:

Mix the almond oil slowly into the granulated sugar. Add the peppermint essential oil. Add drops of pomegranate or raspberry juice. Mix well until color is even throughout.

Citrus Scrub

Ingredients:

Course Sea salt (1 cup)

Raw sugar (1/2 cup)

Coconut oil (1/2 cup)

Sweet orange essential oil (10 drops)

Grapefruit essential oil (10 drops)

Lemon essential oil (5 drops)

Directions:

Combine the sugar and sea salt in a small jar but don't fill to the top.

Heat the coconut oil on low heat until it liquefies

Remove from heat and add all the essential oils

Pour the essential oil mixture and coconut oil over the sugar and sea salt mixture

Do not stir. Apply and massage on the body for some minutes. Rinse

Delectable Scrub

Ingredients:

Organic cane sugar (1 cup)

Celtic sea salt (1/3 cup)

Organic coconut oil (1/2 cup)

Almond oil (2-3 tbsp)

Vitamin E (1 tbsp)

Lavender essential oil (few drops)

Directions:

Combine all ingredients, oils should be last. Mix well. Apply to body.Massage into skin. Rinse

Banana Sugar Scrub

Ingredients:

Banana (1 ripe)

Granulated sugar (3 tablespoons)

Your favorite essential oil (optional)

Directions:

Use a fork to smash ingredients together in a bowl

Do not over- smash so it won't become too thin

Massage mixture all over your body

Rinse off with warm water.

Peppermint/Lavender Foot Scrub

Ingredients:

Salt (1 cup)

Sweet almond oil (1/3 cup)

Peppermint essential oil (10 drops)

Lavender essential oil (5 drops)

Directions:

Combine ingredients thoroughly in a ceramic or glass bowl.

Apply on feet. Leave for a few minutes. Rinse with warm water

Mild Oatmeal Body Scrub

Ingredients:

Finely ground oatmeal (1 cup)

Lavender essential oil (8 drops)

Tangerine essential oil (8 drops)

Rosewood essential oil (8 drops)

Chamomile (4 drops)

Dried lavender petals (1 tbsp, optional)

Directions:

Add oatmeal in a ceramic bowl. Add the essential oils drop by drop. Stir continuously to avoid clumps. Pour in an airtight jar and refrigerate. Combine one tablespoon of the mixture with some water to form a paste. Gently rub onto skin. It can be stored for up to a year.

Body Buffer

Ingredients:

Jojoba Oil (1/4 cup)

Liquid Soap (1/4 cup)

Very Fine Sea Salt (1/2 cup)

Essential Oil (1/2 tsp)

Directions:

In a small bowl, combine all the ingredients and mix thoroughly. Pour into a flip-top bottle. Scrub is in liquid form.

Ginger/ Coconut Oil Sugar Scrub

Ingredients:

Coconut oil (1/4 cup)

Coarsely chopped ginger (1 tbsp)

Carrier oil of choice (1/4 cup)

Granulated sugar (3/4 cup)

Kosher salt (1/4 cup)

Essential oil of choice (1-4 drops)

Directions:

Heat the coconut oil and ginger in a small pan over low heat until liquefied. Remove from heat. Use coffee filter or cheesecloth to press through. Mix warm oils with any carrier oil. Stir in salt and sugar. Add essential oil. Apply to body, massage into skin and rinse.

Ginger/ Orange Foot Scrub

Ingredients:

Brown sugar (1 cup)

Sweet almond oil (1/3 cup)

Orange essential oil (12 drops)

Ginger essential oil (3drops)

Directions:

Combine ingredients thoroughly in a ceramic or glass bowl. Apply on feet. Leave for a few minutes. Rinse with warm water

Gentle Magnesium Foot Scrub

Ingredients:

Epsom salt (1 cup)

Olive oil (¼ cup)

Liquid castile soap (1 teaspoon)

Essential oils (10-15 drops)

Directions:

Mix all ingredients in a small bowl. Add essential oils until desired scent is achieved. Store in airtight jar Use a teaspoon sized quantity to exfoliate feet as needed. Rinse after use.

Cinnamon/ Orange Coffee Scrub Recipe

Ground coffee (1 cup)

Salt (1 tbsp)

Ground cinnamon (1 tsp)

Sweet almond oil (1/3 cup)

Grapefruit essential oil (8 drops)

Orange (8 drops)

Peppermint (4 drops)

Directions:

Mix salt, coffee and essential oils in a glass bowl. Slowly add almond oil slowly and stir continuously until the mixture attains moist sand consistency.

Spicy Sugar Scrub (for Men and Women)

Ingredients:

Organic brown sugar (1 cup)

White granulated sugar (1 cup)

Hazelnut, macadamia nut, almond or soybeans base oil (¾ cup)

Powdered cinnamon (2 tsp)

Powdered ginger (2 tsp)

Powdered nutmeg (2 tsp)

Essential oils (40 drops of any three different types that is good for your skin)

Directions:

Combine all the ingredients except the essential oil in a medium-sized bowl.

Use a whisk to blend all ingredients thoroughly

Add essential oil drop by drop. Blend after each addition.

Spoon mixture into a storage jar with a tight-fitting lid.

Using circular motions, massage ½ cup of scrub onto skin

Rinse.

Exfoliating Sugar Scrub

Ingredients:

White sugar (28g)

Jojoba or Fractionated Coconut Oil (28 mls)

Vegetable Glycerin (5 tsp)

Liquid Castile Soap (28 mls)

Vitamin E Oil (1/2 tsp)

Essential Oil (25 drops)

Directions:

Pour the sugar into a small mixing bowl.

Add the castile soap, oils and glycerin to the sugar.

Mix well.

Add the essential oil and again mix well.

Spoon scrub into a clean tight fitting jar.

BODY LOTIONS, CREAMS & OILS RECIPES

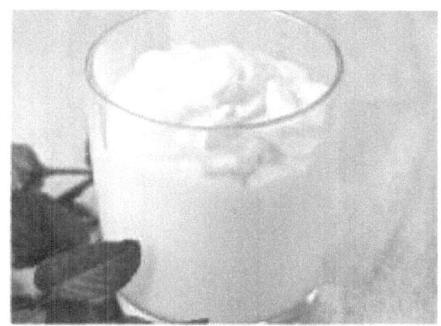

Easy Lotion

Ingredients:

Olive oil (1 cup)

Coconut oil (8 tbsp)

Beeswax, pastilles (8 tbs)

Vitamin E oil (1/2 tsp)

Essential oil (20 drops

Directions:

Combine beeswax pastilles, olive oil and coconut oil in a jar

Put the jar into a saucepan and then fill the saucepan with water, ¾ way up the jar.

(Be careful, the water mustn't get into the oil mixture)

Heat and stir on the stove over low heat until it melts.

Leave to cool at room temperature or refrigerated.

Add in the essential oil and Vitamin E

While it's cooling, use a fork to stir thoroughly every 15 minutes.

Non-Greasy Homemade Moisturizing Lotion

Ingredients:

Aloe Vera gel (1 cup)

Vitamin E oil (1 tsp)

Grated beeswax (1½ tbsp)

Almond or grape-seed oil (1/2 cup)

Cocoa butter (optional, 1 tbs.)

Essential oils of choice (10 drops)

Directions:

Melt beeswax and oils in a double boiler over low heat.

Combine aloe Vera gel and vitamin E oil in a medium-sized bowl.

Pour the melted oils into a blender. Leave to cool at room temperature.

Once cooled, add the essential oils, put the blender on low speed and slowly pour in the aloe Vera mixture.

Blend the mixture until it looks and feel like lotion.

Pour the lotion into clean jars

Last 6 weeks when refrigerated, less without.

Beeswax Hand Cream

Ingredients:

Beeswax (¼ cup)

Almond oil (¼ cup)

Honey (¼ cup)

Bee pollen (1 tbsp)

Vaseline petroleum jelly (¼ cup)

Glycerin (¼ cup)

Liquid lecithin (2 tbsp)

Lavender essential oil (3 drops)

Directions:

In a double boiler, melt the petroleum jelly and beeswax together.

Add the rest of the ingredients except essential oil and heat for 5 minutes until smooth.

Remove from heat and add the essential oil

While still hot, pour into a jar. It will harden as it cools.

Makes about 1¼ cups.

Coco Beeswax Hand Cream

Ingredients:

Beeswax (¼ cup)

Baby oil (3 tbsp)

Coconut oil (¼ cup)

Rosewood essential oil (3drops)

Glycerin (1/3 cup)

Directions:

In a double boiler, melt the coconut oil and beeswax together.

Add the rest of the ingredients, except essential oil and heat for 5 minutes until smooth.

Remove from heat and add the essential oil

While still hot, pour into a jar. It will harden as it cools.

Makes about 1 cup.

Bee Pollen Hand Cream

Ingredients:

Petroleum Jelly (1/2 cup)

Glycerin (1/2 Cup)

Beeswax (1/3 cup)

Bee pollen (2 tablespoons)

Lavender essential oil (3drops)

Directions:

In a double boiler, melt the petroleum jelly and beeswax together.

Add the glycerin and then heat for a few minutes until the mixture is well heated.

Add the bee pollen and essential oil.

While still hot, pour into a jar. It will harden as it cools.

Makes about 1¼ cups

Beeswax Cold Cream

Ingredients:

Beeswax (1/3 cup)

Glycerin (¼ cup)

Liquid lecithin (1 tbsp)

Baby oil (¼ cup)

Almond oil (¼ cup)

Bee pollen (1 tbsp)

Essential oil of choice (3drops)

Directions:

Melt beeswax over a double boiler.

Add the rest of the ingredients, except essential oil and heat until smooth.

Add the essential oil

While still hot, pour into a container. It will harden as it cools.

Makes about 1½ cups

Beeswax Almond Hand Cream

Ingredients:

Beeswax (¼ cup)

Almond oil (½ cup)

Coconut oil (½ cup)

Rosewater (¼ cup)

Essential oil of choice (3drops)

Directions:

Melt the coconut oil and beeswax over a double boiler. Add the remaining ingredients

Add the rest of the ingredients, except essential oil and heat until smooth.

Add the essential oil

While still hot, pour into a container. It will harden as it cools.

Makes about 1½ cups

Stretch Mark Oil

Ingredients:

Rose (4 drops)

Rosemary (1 drop)

Camellia Oil (1/2 teaspoon)

Sesame Oil (1/2 teaspoon)

Vitamin E Oil (1/2 teaspoon)

Wheat Germ Oil (1/2 teaspoon)

Directions:

Massage on stretch mark areas.

Lush Body Oil

Ingredients:

Sunflower Oil (4 oz)

Hazelnut Nut Oil (1 tsp)

Evening of Primrose Oil (1 tsp)

Macadamia Nut Oil (1 tsp)

Vitamin E Oil--20 drops

Directions:

Mix all ingredients together. Store in tightly covered bottle. Refrigerate for longer shelf life.

Anti-Wrinkle Oil

Ingredients:

Rose (2 drops)

Rosemary (1 drop)

Rosewood (2 drop)

Sandalwood (3 drops)

Directions:

Mix together and apply as needed.

Spot Beater Oil

Ingredients:

Castor Oil (1 oz)

Emu Oil (0.5 oz)

Tea Tree EO (30 drops)

Directions:

Mix together and then package.

Oil easily soaks into skin.

Moisturizing Anti-Aging Face Cream

Ingredients:

Beeswax (4 tsp)

Olive oil (4 tbsp)

Shea butter, coconut oil or mango butter (2tbsp)

Water or green tea (8 tbsp)

Jojoba (1 tbsp)

Glycerin (1 tbsp)

Essential oil (10 to 15 drops)

Directions:

Melt the beeswax and oil in a double boiler. Stir until well mixed. Add the shear butter; stir until it well melted into the wax.

Remove from the heat and then whip with a hand-held mixer while adding the aloe Vera, green tea and glycerin.

Continue whipping until the cream becomes light and fluffy. Leave it to cool to room temperature.

Blend in the essential oil, stir until fully combined. Pour into a container and seal. This recipe makes about 227g of anti-aging face cream.

Note:

Since this recipe contains no preservative, keep unused cream refrigerated for about 6 months. Alternatively, keep in a cool place for about 3 months.

Remove cream from container, using washable or cosmetic spatulas and not your fingers to prevent contamination.

Foot Lotion For Aching Feet

Ingredients:

Almond oil (1 tbsp)

Olive oil (1 tbsp)

Wheat germ oil (1 tbsp)

Eucalyptus essential oil (12 drops)

Directions:

Combine all ingredients in a bottle. Shake thoroughly. Just rub into the heels and feet. Store in a cool dry place.

Dry Hand Lotion

Ingredients:

Unscented Lotion (8 oz)

Patchouli (20 drops)

Sandalwood (40 drops)

Borage (20 drops)

Carrot Tissue (5 drops)

Directions:

Pour the lotion into a bowl.

Add the oils and mix thoroughly.

Put the lotion back into the bottle.

Heavy Duty Hand Cream

Ingredients:

Shaved beeswax (2 Tbsp)

Carnauba wax (1/2 tsp)

Jojoba oil 2 (tbsp)

Aloe Vera gel (1 tsp)

Vitamin E oil (10 drops) or Vitamin E capsules (4)

Any essential oil (1 drop)

Directions:

Melt the beeswax, carnauba wax, Jojoba oil and Aloe Vera in a pot either on the stove or in the microwave.

Remove from heat, beat until cool and add Vitamin E oil before the mixture thickens.

Continue beating until mixture becomes creamy.

Add essential oil and keep beating until cream has totally cooled.

Spoon cream into a jar and store in a cool dark place

Lemon Facial Cleansing Cream

Ingredients:

Beeswax (1 tbsp)

Jojoba oil or Coconut oil (3 tbsp)

Witch hazel (1 tbsp)

Lemon juice (1 tbsp)

Bicarbonate of soda 1/8 tsp. (basically a pinch)

Lemon essential oil (6 drops)

Directions:

In a saucepan, melt the beeswax over low heat.

Add the coconut oil (or jojoba) and beat for 5 minutes with a hand mixer.

Heat the witch hazel and lemon juice in another saucepan until warm.

Add in the bicarbonate of soda to dissolve.

Add this liquid mixture to the cream, beat until well combined.

Leave the cream to cool for a while

Add the lemon essential oil.

Spoon into a container.

PERFUMES RECIPES

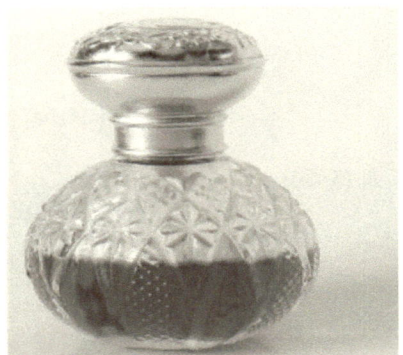

Oriental Nights Perfume

Ingredients:

Sandalwood (4 drops)

Musk (4 drops)

Frankincense (3 drops)

Jojoba oil (2 teaspoons)

Directions:

Combine all the ingredients together.

Shake well. Allow to settle for 12 hours.

Store in a cool dry area.

Whispering Drops Perfume

Ingredients:

Distilled water (2 cups)

Vodka 3 (tbsp)

Sandalwood essential oil (5 drops)

Bergamot essential oil (10 drops)

Cassis essential oil (10 drops)

Directions:

Combine all the ingredients together.

Shake well. Allow to settle for 12 hours

Store in a cool dry area.

Relaxing Summer Body Spray

Ingredients:

Witch hazel (1 tbsp)

Lemon Extract (1 tbsp)

Cucumber Extract (1 tbsp)

Water (1 cup)

Directions:

Combine all ingredients

Transfer to a pump spray bottle

Citrus Bloom Body Splash

Ingredients:

Distilled water (2 cups)

Vodka (3 tbsp)

Finely chopped orange and lemon peel (1tablespoon each)

Lemon verbena essential oil (5 drops)

Mandarin essential oil (10 drops)

Orange essential oil (10 drops)

Directions:

Add the fruit peels with the vodka in a jar. Cover and leave for a week. Strain the liquid and then add the water and essential oils to the liquid. Leave for 2 weeks but shake the jar once a day. Keep in a cool dark area.

Soothing Body Perfume

Ingredients:

Sandalwood (25 drops Base note)

Rose, Jasmine or Neroli (3 drops of Middle note)

Jojoba (2 tbsp)

Directions:

Blend all the oils together. Store in an airtight dark-colored glass jar. Leave for some days to mature. Dab only a drop onto your pulse points. Use sparingly due to the heavy concentration of essential oils.

BOOK 2

100 Plus Simple Homemade Organic Body Scrub Recipes

For Face And Body Exfoliating

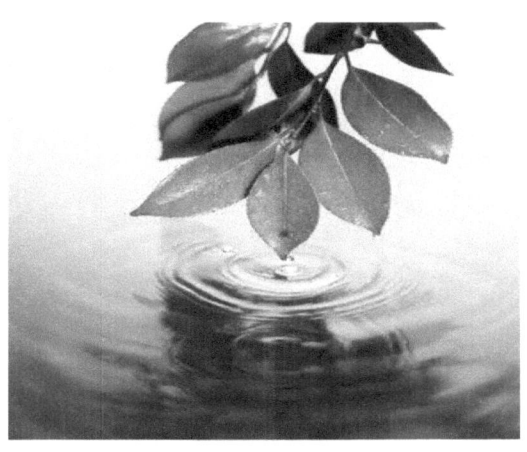

INTRODUCTION

I love my skin. That is because it is soft and so smooth. The secret is that I exfoliate regularly.

Our skin is a living organ. It breathes and lives and requires a lot of care much more than any other organ in the body. Let's not forget the role it also plays in protecting us from the elements.

Exfoliating is the primary treatment for your skin. It is simply the process of getting rid of the dead skin cells that are on the skin's surface and when these dead skin cells are taken off, the healthier and younger looking skin resurfaces.

If you want to have a radiant and smooth skin, exfoliating is a must. Failure to exfoliate leaves your skin covered with dead cells that muck up the surface and gives you a dull and older look. When you repeatedly ignore this process, foundation applied won't smooth over your skin cleanly. Moisturizers won't soak in properly either. Exfoliating should be a vital part of our day to day beauty routine.

Facial scrub is important for breaking white -heads, cleansing the skin and dislodging build-up in the pores. It smoothens and refines the texture of the skin. It enhances blood flow to the body as well.

How Often Should You Exfoliate?

Most health professionals say that two times a week is sufficient. For people with sensitive skin, less is required. Do not scrub too hard and too often if you have a sensitive skin otherwise you will end up removing healthy cells and your skin will look red and feel sore. Simply rub the particles firmly but gently in circular motions. Too much exfoliation will irritate the skin.

Women with oily skin need to exfoliate more frequently than women with dry skin. However, if your skin becomes irritated or dry after exfoliation, you shouldn't scrub so hard. Simply reduce how often you exfoliate. It might just be that you are allergic to the products you used.

Use exfoliating cleansers that contain sugar, sea salt, walnuts, ground almonds, seeds or other grainy components.

Exfoliating The Entire Body

While it is good to exfoliate the face, the entire body needs to receive similar treatment. This is because the skin sheds up to 50,000 dead cells per minute. Not all dead cells fall off; some of them simply build up to clog pores or leave you with a rough skin.

Exfoliate your arms, neck, back, chest and back to prevent body acne. When you exfoliate, the dead skin cells that are in the parts of the body where you've waxed or shaved will be prevented from plugging up follicles. It can even out skin tone and keeps your skin soft and hydrated.

Procedure:

Wet your body in the shower from head to toe.

Start with the soles of your feet and work your way up your body.

Remove rough spots and calluses on your feet using a pumice stone. If you have very rough feet, add a cup of milt to a basin of warm water, stir and soak your feet inside it for 30 minutes before entering the shower.

Apply your scrub to your gloves or loofah. Scrub your body in a circular motion beginning with the bottoms and work your way up. Don't scrub too hard when you get to the bikini area because of the sensitive nature of the skin.

Use a body brush to scrub your back and those places that cannot easily be reached.

Scrub your face gently. Pay attention to your mouth and eyes but you must use an exfoliating product meant for the face because it is gently that those made for the body.

Remember your hands; they should look and feel soft too.

Rinse your body using lukewarm water

Step out of the shower

Pat your face dry with a clean towel after exfoliating.

Apply a moisturizing lotion all over your body

Ensure you use facial moisturizers and body lotions that contain alpha or beta hydroxy acids because they help in removing dead skin cells.

Tips:

After exfoliating, apply sunscreen if you are going out in the sun. You do not want the fresh skin to be damaged by the sun especially since it may be slightly irritated.

Preserve the smoothness and avoid breakouts by using a non-comedogenic moisturizer

Don't scrub your face too hard, this can cause damage to and hurt your skin.

Do not exfoliate if you have an open wound or cut or if you are sunburned.

Although a variety of body scrubs are available on the market these days. They are filled with addictives and preservatives that could harm your skin in the long run. It is advisable to be cautious of what we absorb into our skin. It is unrealistic to eat organic foods and then introduce chemicals into our bodies through our skin. The solution to a wonderful skin is in your kitchen, not the store!

The Double Boiler Method

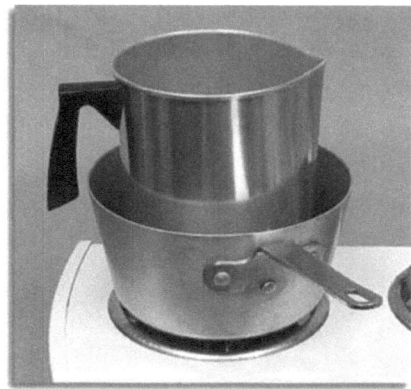

Some of the recipes in this book require the use of the double boiler method to make.

A double boiler method is effective for heating materials gently without scorching or burning them. You may either buy one but they are quite simply to make on your own.

Get two pots, the smaller one should fit into the big one.

Fill the big pot with some water.

Place a one inch high sheet metal ring into the big pot. This will help the small pot to sit perfectly.

Place the small pot on top of the big pot of water. It should not touch the water.

As the water boils, the heat will be transferred to the smaller pot which has been filled with whatever you want to melt or cook.

This can either be done in the oven or on the stove

The recipes in this book are great and incredibly amazing. You will even be tempted to eat them!

I have used organic ingredients and created recipes that you will definitely love. They are tested and proven. It is my belief that you will enjoy using them as much as I have.

Essential Oils

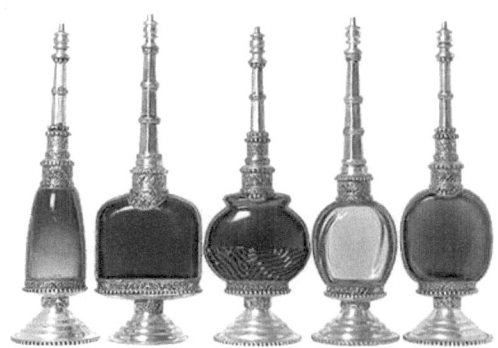

Essential oils are aromatic oils popularly used in the cosmetic industry. They are highly concentrated and have rejuvenating and healing abilities –the best treatment for your skin. These oils are extracted from the leaves, flowers, stem, seeds and roots of plants, the bark of trees as well as the peel of citrus fruits. They do not dissolve in Aloe Vera juice or water but dissolve only a little in vinegar.

If wrongly used, essential oils are harmful and this is the reason they must be kept out of children's reach. They are flammable as well and should never be placed near fires.

Essential oil should be stored in a dry and cool place. This enables it to retain its potency for 5 to 10 years. The citrus oils are an exception, however, because it only retains its healing properties for 6 to 12 months.

Be familiar with the properties and contraindications of every essential oil before using it.

Safety Tips To Remember When Preparing Your Own Body Scrubs:

Undiluted essential oils must never be directly applied to the skin.

They should not be taken internally because they are highly concentrated and toxic if ingested.

Some essential oils may cause allergic reactions and skin irritation.

Some essential oils are not suitable for pregnant women and individuals with health conditions like asthma and epilepsy.

Essential oils like citrus oils and bergamot may cause skin sensitivity to sunlight, even when diluted. They should not be applied on sunny or extremely hot days.

If the oil accidentally gets into your nose or eyes while working with it, flush out the affected part immediately using unscented fatty oil like olive, soybean, almond or peanut.

To determine possible allergic reactions of a particular oil, carry out a skin patch test. Mix one or two drops of the essential oil and ½ to 1 teaspoon of base oil in a small bowl.

Dab a small portion in the inside of your elbow, behind your ear, inside your upper arm, or behind your knee. Cover it for 24 hours with a band aid. If no irritation occurs, then the oil is safe to use.

Below are a few essential oils that are widely used in cosmetics. You can be creative and add to the under-listed to create your own unique blend.

Lemon and Bergamot should not be used on sensitive skin.

Lasmine, Chamomile, Rose and Geranium should not be used during pregnancy.

Eucalyptus, Frankincense, Lavender, Neroli, Palmarosa, Petitgrain, Orange, Rosewood, Sandalwood, Ylang Ylang.

Base Oils

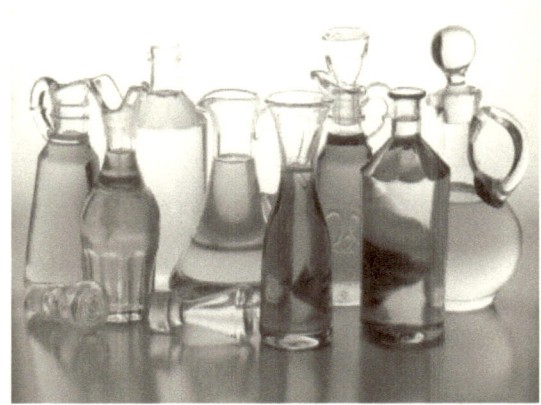

Base oils (also known as carrier oils) are primarily used in diluting essential oils before applying them to the skin. They are derived from fruits, vegetables, beans, seeds and nuts. They are generally cold-pressed vegetable oils without their own scent and this is why they can serve as perfect counterparts for essential oils.

Grapeseed, Jojoba, Sunflower, Sweet Almond, Avocado Peanut, Sesame and Apricot kernel are examples of a few of them.

Organically grown base oils which have been extracted naturally and processed minimally are the best for personal care recipes. These particular oils have not been exposed to very high temperatures, bleaching, deodorizing or chemical extraction procedures that can alter or destroy antioxidant properties, natural aromas, flavors and beneficial vitamins.

Check the labels for keywords like *cold-pressed, expeller pressed* or *refined* before you buy.

Remember to always check the expiry date on the bottle and return immediately if the oil is bad. Ensure you make your purchase from reliable retailers that have a high inventory turnover.

Skin professionals sometimes use the terms slide and slip to describe the way oil product glides onto the skin. It indicates that the oil is neither rapidly absorbed nor sticky. This is the kind of base oil that is just right to use as a face or body massage oil. Soybeans oils and organic almond have thinner texture and are therefore excellent massage base oils. Jojoba oil also serves as balancing body oil.

Unlike essential oils, carrier oils have a short shelf life and becomes rancid once opened.

Fragrance Oils

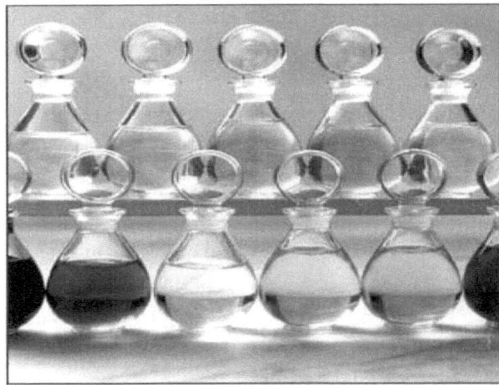

Fragrance oils, also called aroma oils, flavor oils or aromatic oils are natural essential oils that have been diluted with a carrier like mineral oil, vegetable oil or propylene glycol.

Fragrance oils are used to add a variety of scent to those fruits that do not produce essential oil such as mango, strawberry and watermelon. It is possible to even make one that will smell like chocolate! They serve as a fantastic fragrant addition to body scrubs and lotions.

However, before using these aromatics, be sure to read and follow the instructions provided on the label. And like essential oils, only a few drops are required to produce wonderful fragrant results.

Butters – Shea, Cocoa, Mango

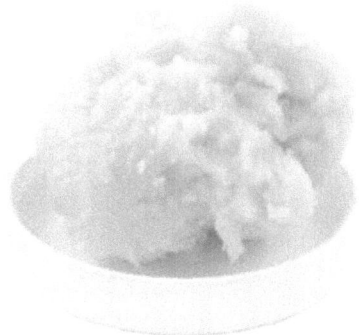

Shea nut butter is ivory-colored. It is a natural fat extraction from the fruit of the Shea tree. This fruit is called a nut and has an avocado-like seed in it. It is from this seed that Shea butter is extracted. Its uses are diverse.

It has soothing and moisturizing effects.

It prevents certain sun allergies.

It protects the skin from harmful UV rays.

It helps capillary circulation and cell regeneration.

Cocoa Butter is an aromatic solid butter from the seeds of the cacao tree which is extracted and roasted. This solid butter softens at body temperature. It adds a thick, rich and creamy consistency to body scrubs, lotions, creams and soaps which improves the skin's elasticity by helping to reduce dryness.

Mango Butter is cold pressed and rendered from the mango tree's seed kernel. It works effectively as a mild lubricant for the skin and has beneficial moisturizing properties. It is an excellent quality base ingredient perfect for body care products. It is also loaded with essential fatty acids.

SUGAR BODY SCRUB RECIPES

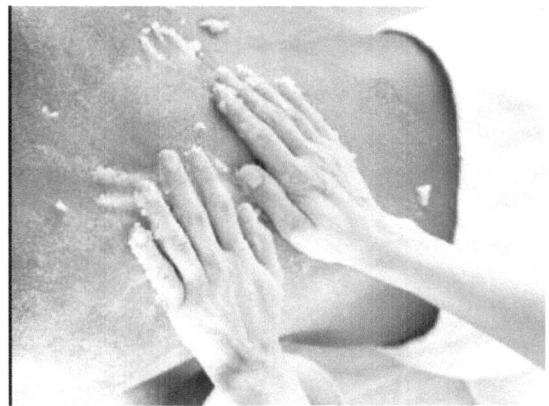

Sugar scrubs are highly recommended for individuals who have sensitive skin. They are gentler than salt and remove dead skin cells, dirt and toxin leaving the skin with a healthy and revitalized glow.

Sugar has anti-aging properties because it produces an alpha hydroxy acid known as glycolic acid which has been proven by generations to rejuvenate skin. Sugar scrubs give your skin a natural appearance and a younger glow.

Mango Colada

Ingredients:

Coconut oil (1/2 teaspoon)

Coconut fragrance oil (1/4 teaspoon)

Mango fragrance oil (1/4 teaspoon)

Pineapple fragrance oil (1/4 teaspoon)

Organic white sugar (1 cup)

Directions:

Mix oils into plastic bowl or glass

Add sugar and mix thoroughly until well blended.

Shelf Life: Store in a tightly sealed container for about a month.

Orange Sunrise

Ingredients:

Melted cocoa butter (2 tablespoons)

Warmed olive oil (4 tablespoons)

Orange juice (4 tablespoons)

Essential orange oil (2 drops)

Organic brown sugar (1 cup)

Directions:

Blend all the ingredients with a blender until fluffy and light.

Blend again if the mixture separates.

Shelf life: Store in a jar or a tightly-capped bottle. Refrigerate for up to 2 weeks.

Sweet Avocado

Ingredients:

Almond oil (5 drops)

Ripe avocado (1)

Organic white sugar (3/4 cup)

Directions:

Blend almond oil and pour into avocado. Add sugar and use a hand held blender to mix until smooth.

Shelf life: Use immediately.

Jasmine Rose

Ingredients:

Grape- seed oil (10 teaspoon)

Patchouli essential oil (7 drops)

Jasmine essential oil (4 drops)

Rose essential oil (2 drops)

Organic white sugar (1 cup)

Directions:

Combine all the ingredients in a bowl.

Shelf Life: Store for up to 6 months in an air tight container.

Grape Soufflé

Ingredients:

Green grapes (1 cup)

Honey (1 teaspoon)

Egg yolk (1)

Organic white (1 cup)

Directions:

Crush green grapes to pulp. Add egg yolk and honey. Use a hand mixer to whip together

Shelf Life: Store for 24 hours in an air tight container.

Chamomile Petitgrain

Ingredients:

Chamomile essential oil (3 drops)

Petitgrain essential oil (2 drops)

Organic brown sugar (1 cup)

Dried chamomile flowers (1/4 cup)

Directions:

Combine all the ingredients in a bowl.

Shelf Life: Store for up to a month in an air tight container.

Violet Vibrations

Ingredients:

Coconut oil (2 ounces)

Violet fragrant oil (4 drops)

Organic white sugar (1/2 cup)

Red food coloring (optional, 1 drop)

Blue food coloring (optional, 1 drop)

Directions:

Mix ingredients together. Shelf life: Store for up to a month in an air tight container.

Sugar And Spice

Ingredients:

Baking soda (1/2 cup)

Organic white sugar (2 tablespoons)

Organic ground cinnamon (1 teaspoon)

Organic ground ginger (1/2 teaspoon)

Organic ground cloves (1/4 teaspoon)

Almond oil (2 tablespoons)

Directions:

Combine the dry ingredients in a bowl. Then, add the almond oil. Mix them all together until well blended. Shelf Life: Store for up to a month in an air tight container.

Apricot Honey Butter

Ingredients:

Kernel oil (10 oz apricot)

Cocoa butter (2 oz)

Organic brown sugar (1 cup)

Organic honey (1 tablespoon)

Directions:

Heat the cocoa butter in the double boiler top until it is melted. Remove from heat and add the rest of the ingredients. Beat with a wooden spoon till it is smooth and cooled. Shelf life: Put in a glass jar, close tightly and refrigerate for 1 month.

Jasmine And Aloe

Ingredients:

Apricot kernel oil (1/4 cup)

Cocoa butter (1 teaspoon)

Coconut oil (1 teaspoon)

Aloe Vera gel (1 teaspoon)

Jasmine fragrance oil (5 drops)

Organic brown sugar (1 cup)

Directions:

Combine ingredients into a bowl and mix thoroughly. Shelf life: Store in glass jar for up to one month.

Brown Sugar And Almond

Ingredients:

Ground almonds (1 handful)

Brown sugar (2 tablespoons)

Honey (2 tablespoons)

Directions:

Squash almonds in a food processor. Add egg yolk and honey. Use a hand mixer and whip together.

Shelf Life: Store for up to 1 week in an air tight container

Green Tea and Honey

Ingredients:

Honey (2 tablespoons)

Green tea bag (1 organic)

White sugar (1 cup organic)

Almond oil (2 tablespoons)

Directions:

Place sugar in a medium sized mixing bowl. Tear open green tea bag and add to it. Stir to combine.

Next, add the almond oil and mix. Lastly, add 1 tablespoon of honey at a time and mix well.

Shelf life: Refrigerate and use within 1 week.

Spring Fever

Ingredients:

Frankincense essential oil (3 drops)

Lime essential oil (2 drops)

Rose essential oil (2 drops)

Organic white sugar (1 cup)

Directions:

Mix ingredients together in a large bowl.

Shelf Life: Store for up to 6 months in an air tight container.

Sandalwood Rose

Ingredients:

Rose essential oil (2 drops)

Sandalwood essential oil (5 drops)

Ylang Ylang essential oil (2 drops)

Organic brown sugar (1 cup)

Directions:

Combine ingredients in a bowl.

Shelf Life: Store for up to 6 months in an air tight container.

Wheat and Oats

Ingredients:

Organic white sugar (1/2 cup)

Olive oil (2 teaspoons)

Rolled oats (1/4)

Wheat germ (1/4)

Directions:

Mix ingredients together in a large bowl.

Shelf Life: Store for up to 1 month in an air tight container

Grapefruit and Sugar

Ingredients:

Organic brown sugar (1/2 cup)

Sunflower oil (2 teaspoons)

Organic white sugar (1/2)

Vitamin E (1/2 teaspoon)

Grapefruit essential oil (3 drops)

Directions:

Mix ingredients together in a large bowl.

Shelf Life: Store for up to a day in an air tight container.

Herb

Ingredients:

Honey (1/4 cup)

Dry sage (1 teaspoon)

Dry thyme (1 teaspoon)

Dry rosemary (1 teaspoon)

Organic white sugar (1 cup)

Directions:

Combine ingredients and store.

Shelf Life: Store for up to a week in a sterilized glass jar.

Vanilla Almond

Ingredients:

Whole almonds (1/3 cup)

Almond oil (1 tablespoon)

Vanilla fragrance oil (1/8 teaspoon)

Organic white sugar (1 cup)

Directions:

Pour almonds into a food processor or chopper. Then chop till particles are fine.

Combine with the sugar and oils.

Shelf Life: Store in a tightly sealed container. It lasts for up to 2 months

Vanilla Patchouli

Ingredients:

Organic brown sugar (1 cup)

Vanilla fragrance oil (20 drops)

Patchouli essential oil (5 drops)

Ylang-ylang essential oil (5 drops)

Directions:

Mix ingredients together in a large bowl.

Shelf Life: Store for up to 6 months in an air tight container.

Pineapple Passions

Ingredients:

Ripe pineapple (1 cup)

Organic white sugar (1 cup)

Passionflower oil (3 drops)

Sunflower oil (1 tablespoon)

Directions:

Puree cucumber in blender. Then add oils to a mixing bowl of sugar. Mix thoroughly.

Shelf Life: Store for up to 1 week in an air tight container

Cucumber Ylang Ylang

Ingredients:

Ripe cucumber (1)

Organic white sugar (1 cup)

Ylang Ylang essential oil (2 drops)

Sunflower oil (1 tablespoon)

Directions:

Puree cucumber in blender. Next add oils to a mixing bowl of sugar. Mix thoroughly.

Shelf Life: Store for up to a week in an air tight container.

Bergamot Neroli

Ingredients:

Organic white sugar (2 ½ cups)

Almond oil (1/2 cup)

Shea butter (1 tablespoon)

Bergamot essential oil (2 drops)

Neroli essential oil (1 drop)

Directions:

Combine the almond oil and sugar in a large bowl and mix well. Then add the Shea butter and whip/ mix/ with a hand held blender on high speed for about 3minutes. You will have a grainy paste.Shelf Life: Store in a tightly sealed container for up to 2 months

Strawberry Banana Bliss

Ingredients:

Banana (1 ripe)

Pineapples (1/4 cup)

Strawberries (1/4 cup)

Apricot kernel oil (2 tablespoons)

Organic white sugar (1 cup)

Directions:

Puree fruit in a blender. Mix fruit with sugar and oil. Shelf Life: Store for up to 3 days in an air tight container.

Tea Tree Temptations

Ingredients:

Sunflower oil (8 teaspoons)

Jasmine oil (6 drops)

Tea tree oil (2 drops)

Neroli oil (2 drops)

Organic white sugar (1 cup)

Directions:

Mix ingredients together in a glass jar.

Shelf Life: Store for up to 2 months in an air tight container.

Fresca

Ingredients:

Tangerine fragrance oil (7 drops)

Lemon essential oil (4 drops)

Organic white sugar (1 cup)

Directions:

Combine ingredients in a bowl.

Shelf Life: Store for up to 6 months in an air tight container.

Snow In The Summertime

Ingredients:

Sugar (1/2 cup)

Olive oil (2 teaspoons)

Heavy whipping cream (1/4 cup)

Directions:

Mix ingredients together in a large bowl and use a hand mixer to mix till light.

Shelf Life: Store for up to a day in an air tight container

Maya Papaya

Ingredients:

Papaya (1/2)

Lemon or lime juice (1/2 teaspoon)

Honey (1 teaspoon)

Organic white sugar (1 cup)

Directions:

Puree papaya in a blender. Next, add lemon juice to papaya and blend again. Add the honey and papaya to the sugar in mixing bowl. Mix well

Shelf Life: Store for up to a day in an air tight container.

Cinnamon Celebration

Ingredients:

Organic white sugar (1/2 cup)

Ground cinnamon (1/2 teaspoon)

Almond oil (1 tablespoon)

Organic brown sugar (1/2 cup)

Directions:

Combine sugars and cinnamon. Add oils and mix thoroughly.

Shelf Life: Store for up to a month in an air tight container.

Sweet Plum

Ingredients:

Plums (6)

Almond oil (1 teaspoon)

Organic brown sugar (1 cup)

Directions:

Puree the plums in a blender. Add almond oil and plums to sugar.

Shelf Life: Use immediately.

Neroli Lemon Grass

Ingredients:

Lemongrass oil (2 drops)

Neroli oil (2 drops)

Organic brown sugar (1/2 cup)

Directions:

Combine the ingredients in a bowl and mix thoroughly.

Shelf Life: Store for up to 6 months in an air tight container

Peach Meringue

Ingredients:

Peach (1 ripe)

Egg white (1)

Organic white sugar (1 cup)

Directions:

Purée the peach in a blender. Next, beat the egg white until stiff and then fold the peach purée into the egg white. Add the sugar and stir by hand.

Shelf life: Use immediately.

Vanilla Coconut

Ingredients:

Coconut oil (1 tablespoon)

Jojoba oil (2 tablespoons)

Vanilla fragrance oil (10 drops)

Coconut fragrance oil (10 drops)

Organic white sugar (1 cup)

Directions:

Combine the ingredients in a bowl and mix thoroughly. Shelf Life: Store for up to 6 months in an air tight container

Field of Flowers

Ingredients:

Grapeseed oil (6-8 teaspoon)

Chamomile oil (2 drops)

Rose oil (2 drops)

Geranium oil (2 drops)

Jasmine oil (2 drops)

Organic white sugar (1 cup)

Directions:

Add oils to a mixing bowl of sugar. Mix thoroughly. Shelf Life: Store for up to 1 week in an air tight container.

Lavender Apricot

Ingredients:

Organic white sugar (1/2 cup)

Plain yogurt (1/4 cup)

Mashed fresh apricots (1/8 cup)

Honey (1/8 cup)

Lavender essential oils (2 drops)

Directions:

Mix ingredients together in a large bowl.

Shelf Life: Store for 1 day in an air tight container.

Strawberry Daiquiri

Ingredients:

Very ripe fresh strawberries (1/2 cup)

Organic white sugar (1 cup)

Strawberry fragrance oil (2 drops)

Directions:

Puree strawberries and add fragrance oil and sugar.

Shelf Life: Store for a day in an air tight container.

Sweet Sage And Lemon

Ingredients:

Fresh sage (2 tablespoons)

Almond oil (4 tablespoons)

Lemon essential oil (2 drops)

Organic white sugar (1 cup)

Directions:

In a food processor, place sage or chop by hand until fine. Add the sugar and sage together in a mixing bowl and stir until sage is evenly distributed. Then add remaining ingredients and stir to mix.

Shelf life: Store and refrigerate for up to a week in an air tight container.

Almond Honey

Ingredients:

Crushed almonds (2 tablespoon)

Honey (1 tablespoon)

Organic brown sugar (1 cup)

Directions:

Place almonds in a food processor and chop until fine. In a mixing bowl, add almonds to remaining ingredients and stir to combine.

Shelf life: Store for up to a week in an air tight container

Lavender Lime

Ingredients:

Lime oil (3 drops)

Lavender oil (3 drops)

Organic white sugar (1 cup)

Directions:

Combine in a bowl and mix thoroughly.

Shelf Life: Store for up to 3 month in an air tight container.

Wheat Germ

Ingredients:

Cocoa butter (1/4 cup)

Organic wheat germ (1 tablespoon)

Apricot kernel oil (1 tablespoon)

Vitamin E oil (1 tablespoon)

Organic brown sugar (1/2)

Directions:

Use the double boiler method to melt the cocoa butter. Pour into a mixing bowl. Next, add remaining ingredients and stir to combine.

Shelf life: Store for up to 1 week in an air tight container.

Lemon Poppy

Ingredients:

Olive oil (1/2 cup)

Poppy seeds (1/2 cup)

Lemon essential oil (1/4 teaspoon)

Organic white sugar (1/2 cup)

Directions:

Thoroughly mix all of the ingredients together.

Shelf Life: Store for 1 month in an air tight container

Apple Honey

Ingredients:

Apple, cored, quartered (1)

Honey (2 tablespoon)

Teaspoon sage (1/2 tablespoon)

Organic white sugar (1 cup)

Directions:

Place the apple slices into a food processor and chop. Then, add honey, sage and sugar.

Shelf life: Use immediately.

Vanilla Rose

Ingredients:

Rosewater (2 tablespoon)

Vanilla fragrance oil (10 drops)

Rose fragrance oil (4 drops)

Organic white sugar (1 cup)

Directions:

Combine ingredients and mix well.

Shelf Life: Store for up to 1 month in an air tight container.

Grapeseed And Grapes

Ingredients:

Grapeseed oil (8 teaspoon)

White grapes (1/2 cup)

Organic white sugar (1 cup)

Directions:

Puree grapes in a blender. Next, add Grapeseed oil, grapes to a mixing bowl of sugar. Mix thoroughly

Shelf Life: Store for up to 3 days in an air tight container

Jojoba Aloe Vera

Ingredients:

Jojoba oil (2 tablespoons)

Cocoa butter (2 tablespoon)

Vitamin E oil (1 tablespoon)

Aloe Vera gel (2 tablespoon)

Organic white sugar (1 cup)

Directions:

Combine in a bowl and mix thoroughly.

Shelf Life:

Store for up to 1 month in an air tight container.

Bananas Forrester

Ingredients:

Ripe banana (1)

Almond oil (1 tablespoon)

Organic white sugar (1/2 cup)

Organic brown sugar (1/2 cup)

Directions:

Puree banana in a blender. Then add sugars and blend till smooth. Pour into a bowl and mix in almond oil.

Shelf Life: Use immediately.

Godiva

Ingredients:

Godiva Chocolates (1 handful)

Organic white sugar (1/4 cup)

Peanut oil (2 tablespoon)

Fresh whole milk (2 tablespoon)

Directions:

Use the double boiler method to melt the chocolate. In a mixing bowl add the milk, sugar and peanut oil. Next, pour in chocolate and mix thoroughly.

Shelf Life: Store for up to 1 week in an air tight container

Honey Mint

Ingredients:

Mint (1 tablespoon)

Oil (1 tablespoon)

Honey (1 tablespoon)

Organic white sugar (1 cup)

Directions:

Finely chop the mint by hand or in a food processor. Add mint to sugars and other ingredients.

Shelf Life: Store for up to 1 month in an air tight container

Grapeseed and Avocado

Ingredients:

Grapeseed oil (8 teaspoon)

Avocado (1 ripe)

Organic white sugar (1 cup)

Directions:

Puree avocado in a blender. Then add grapeseed oil to a mixing bowl of sugar.

Mix thoroughly.

Shelf Life: Store for up to 3 days in an air tight container

Sweet Basil

Ingredients:

Basil oil (1 drop)

Fresh basil (2 tablespoons)

Organic white sugar (1 cup)

Directions:

Finely chop basil in food processor. Put all ingredients and mix well.

Shelf Life: Store for one day in an air tight container.

Citrus Sandalwood

Ingredients:

Safflower oil (10 teaspoon)

Orange blossom oil (5 drops)

Sandalwood oil (2 drops)

Organic brown sugar (1 cup)

Directions:

Mix ingredients together and pour into glass jars.

Shelf Life: Store for up to 3 months in an air tight container

SALT BODY SCRUBS

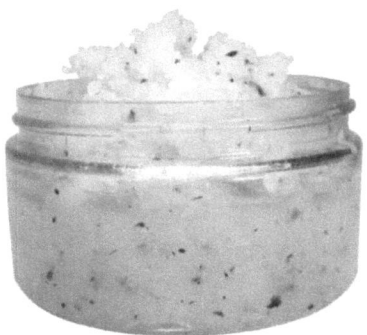

Salt scrubs enhance the circulation to the skin. They are coarser than sugar-based scrubs and have more exfoliating power.

People who have sensitive skin should not use salt scrubs. However, it is best to begin your exfoliating routine once a week.

Chamomile Jasmine

Ingredients:

Dried chamomile leaves (1 tablespoon)

Jasmine essential oil (1 tablespoon)

Crushed organic sea salt (1 cup)

Jojoba oil (3 tablespoon)

Directions:

Combine ingredients in mixing bowl and stir.

Shelf Life: Store for up to 1 week

Geranium

Ingredients:

Crushed organic sea salt (1/2 cup)

Geranium essential oil (4 drops)

Shea butter (2 tablespoons)

Apricot kernel oil (2 tablespoons)

Directions:

Use the double boiler method to melt Shea butter. Add to oils and sea salt

Shelf Life: Store for up to 6 months.

Artichoke

Ingredients:

Fresh artichoke hearts (1)

Canola oil (2 teaspoon)

Crushed organic sea salt (1 cup)

Fresh lemon juice (1 teaspoon)

Directions:

Mash cooked artichoke hearts in a glass bowl and mix with lemon and oil.

Stir well till smooth paste.

Shelf Life: Store for 1 week.

Mucho Mango

Ingredients:

Ripe mango (1)

Mango butter (2 tablespoon)

Crushed organic sea salt (1 cup)

Apricot kernel oil (2 tablespoons)

Directions:

Use the double boiler method to melt mango butter. Puree mango in a blender.

Mix all ingredients in a bowl and stir well.

Shelf Life: Store for 2 months.

Milk And Honey

Ingredients:

Milk or cream (1/4 cup)

Crushed organic sea salt (1 cup)

Honey (1/4 cup)

Directions:

Mix honey and milk (or cream) in an enamel pan or a small glass.

Warm until the honey melts. Remove from heat.

Shelf Life: Store for 1 week.

Cucumber Yogurt

Ingredients:

Cucumber (1 tablespoon)

Parsley (1 tablespoon)

Yogurt (1 tablespoon)

Crushed organic sea salt (1cup)

Directions:

Combine ingredients in mixing bowl and stir.

Almond Milk

Ingredients:

Almond oil (1/4 cup)

1 cup crushed organic sea salt (1 cup)

Almond milk (1/4 cup)

Directions:

Mix ingredients until well mixed.

Shelf Life: Store for 1 week.

Lavender Mint

Ingredients:

Dried lavender (2 tablespoons)

Mint (1 tablespoon)

Crushed organic sea salt (1cup)

Canola oil (4 tablespoons)

Directions:

Place mint on a cutting board and finely chop. Continue with salt, oil and dried lavender.

Shelf Life: Store for 3 months.

Raspberry

Ingredients:

Fresh raspberry (1/2 cup)

1 cup crushed organic sea salt (1 cup)

Sunflower oil (4 tablespoons)

Directions:

Combine ingredients in a food processor.

Shelf Life: Store in a glass jar for a week.

Summer Glow

Ingredients:

Crushed organic sea salt (1/2 cup)

Mango butter (2 tablespoons)

Shea butter (2 tablespoons)

Cocoa butter (2 tablespoons)

Fine silver glitter (1/2 tablespoons)

Directions:

Use the double boiler method to melt all the butters together.

Combine all ingredients in a bowl and use a hand mixer to mix well.

Shelf Life: Store for up to 2 months in an air tight container.

Apricot

Ingredients:

Crushed organic sea salt (1/2 cup)

Fresh apricot (1/2 cup)

Apricot fragrance oil (2 drops)

Directions:

Puree apricot in blender. Mix all ingredients in a bowl and stir well.

Shelf Life: Store for 1 week in an air tight container

Cinnamon And Spice

Ingredients:

Sunflower oil (4 tablespoon)

Crushed organic sea salt (1 cup)

Ground cinnamon (2 tablespoon)

Ground nutmeg (1 tablespoon)

Directions:

Combine ingredients in a bowl and mix thoroughly.

Shelf Life: Store for up to 2 months in an air tight container.

Eucalyptus

Ingredients:

Olive oil (4 tablespoon)

Crushed organic sea salt (1/2 cup)

Eucalyptus essential oil (2 drops)

Directions:

Combine ingredients in a bowl and mix thoroughly.

Shelf Life: Store for up to 6 months in an air tight container.

Milk And Herbs

Ingredients:

Olive oil (4 tablespoon)

Crushed organic sea salt (1/2cup)

Powdered goats milk (2 tablespoon)

Dried thyme (1 tablespoon)

Dried rosemary (1 tablespoon)

Directions:

Combine ingredients in a bowl and mix thoroughly.

Shelf Life: Store for 2 weeks in an air tight container.

Oats And Honey

Ingredients:

Powdered oats (1/4 cup)

Crushed organic sea salt (1/2 cup)

Honey (1/4 cup)

Sweet almond (2 tablespoons)

Directions:

Mix powdered oats and salt. Add the honey and then the oil.

Mix until fully combined.

Shelf Life: Store for 2 months in an air tight container.

Watermelon Splash

Ingredients:

Crushed organic sea salt (1/2 cup)

Fresh watermelon (1/2 cup)

Directions:

Combine ingredients in a bowl and mix well.

Shelf Life: Store for up to 1 week in an air tight container.

Pomegranate

Ingredients:

Apricot kernel oil (4 tablespoon)

Crushed organic sea salt (1 cup)

Pomegranate juice (2 tablespoon)

Pomegranate fragrance oil (3 drop)

Directions:

Combine ingredients in a bowl and mix well.

Shelf Life: Store for up to 2 weeks in an air tight container.

Fruit And Nut

Ingredients:

Crushed almonds (1/2 cup)

Crushed organic sea salt (1/2 cup)

Raisons (2 tablespoons)

Dried cranberries (2)

Almond oil (2 tablespoon)

Directions:

Combine ingredients in a bowl and mix thoroughly.

Shelf Life: Store for 2 months in an air tight container.

Tangerine Mint

Ingredients:

Olive oil (4 tablespoon)

Cup crushed organic sea salt (1/2cup)

Tangerine fragrance oil (2 drops)

Spearmint essential oil (2 drops)

Directions:

Combine all ingredients and mix well.

Shelf Life: Store for up to 6 months in an air tight container.

Ginger Lime

Ingredients:

Crushed organic sea salt (1 cup)

Ground ginger (1 teaspoon)

Fresh lime juice (1 teaspoon)

Macadamia nut oil (4 tablespoon)

Directions:

Combine all ingredients and mix well.

Shelf Life: Store for up to 2 weeks in an air tight container.

Very Berry

Ingredients:

Strawberry fragrance oil (2 drops)

Crushed organic sea salt (1 cup)

Raspberry fragrance oil (2 drops)

Sweet almond oil (2 tablespoon)

Vitamin E oil (2 tablespoon)

Directions:

Combine all the ingredients in a bowl and stir well.

Shelf Life: Store for up to 3 months in a glass jar.

Vanilla Milk

Ingredients:

Vanilla extract (2 tablespoon)

Crushed organic sea salt (1 cup)

Milk (4 tablespoons)

Powdered goat's milk (2 tablespoon)

Directions:

Mix all the ingredients in a glass bowl.

Shelf Life: Store for up to 1 week in a glass jar.

Hazel Nut

Ingredients:

Crushed organic sea salt (1/2 cup)

Hazel nut oil (2 tablespoon)

Crushed hazel nuts (1/4)

Directions:

Mix all ingredients.

Shelf Life: Store for a week in an air tight container.

Tomato Carrot

Ingredients:

Crushed organic sea salt (1/2 cup)

Ripe tomato (1)

Carrot juice (1/4)

Directions:

Puree carrot juice and tomato. Add salt and beat with a hand mixer.

Shelf Life: Store for up to 1 week in an air tight container.

Citrus Blend

Ingredients:

Mango butter (2 tablespoon)

Crushed organic sea salt (1 cup)

Orange essential oil (2 drops)

Lemon essential oil (2 drops)

Grapefruit essential oil (2 drops)

Almond oil (2 tablespoon)

Directions:

Use a double boiler to melt mango butter and add to the other ingredients.

Shelf Life: Store for up to 6 months in an air tight container.

Tangerine

Ingredients:

Tangerine essential oil (2 drop)

Crushed organic sea salt (1 cup)

Dried orange peel powder (4 tablespoons)

Apricot kernel (2 tablespoons)

Directions:

Mix all the ingredients and stir well.

Shelf Life: Store for up to 3 months in a glass jar.

Egyptian Nights

Ingredients:

Crushed organic sea salt (1/2 cup)

Egyptian musk fragrance oil (3 drops)

Epsom salt (1/4 cup)

Directions:

Combine all ingredients and mix well

Shelf Life: Store for up to 6 months in an air tight container.

Frankincense and Sandalwood

Ingredients:

Frankincense essential oil (2 drops)

Crushed organic sea salt (1 cup)

Sandalwood essential oil (2 drops)

Vegetable oil (2 tablespoon)

Directions:

Mix all ingredients in a bowl and stir well.

Shelf Life: Store for up to 3 months in a glass jar.

Rosemary Soy Milk

Ingredients:

Soy milk (2 tablespoon)

Crushed organic sea salt (1 cup)

Dried rosemary (4 tablespoons)

Canola oil (4 tablespoons)

Directions:

Mix all ingredients in a glass bowl.

Shelf Life: Store for up to 1 week in a glass jar.

Pink Champagne

Ingredients:

French pink champagne (2 tablespoon)

Crushed organic sea salt (1 cup)

Epsom salt (2 tablespoon)

Directions:

Mix all ingredients in a glass bowl.

Shelf Life: Store for up to 2 weeks in a glass jar.

Banana Berry

Ingredients:

Ripe banana (1)

Strawberry fragrance oil (3 drops)

Crushed organic sea salt (1/2 cup)

Fresh strawberries (1/4)

Directions:

Combine all ingredients and mix with a hand mixer.

Shelf Life: Store for 2 days in an air tight container

Buttermilk

Ingredients:

Crushed organic sea salt (1/2 cup)

Lemon tea tree essential oil (1 teaspoon)

Buttermilk (2 teaspoon)

Yogurt (2 teaspoons)

Directions:

Mix all ingredients in a mixing bowl.

Shelf Life: Store for a week in an air tight container.

Autumn Harvest

Ingredients:

Peach fragrance oil (3 drops)

Bergamot Essential Oil (3 drops)

Vanilla Essential Oil (3 drops)

Range fragrance oil (3 drops)

Crushed organic sea salt (1/2 cup)

Directions:

Combine all ingredients and mix.

Shelf Life: Store for up to 6 months in an air tight container.

Rose Bouquet

Ingredients:

Pink Rose Petal Powder (2 tablespoon)

Crushed organic sea salt (1 cup)

Rose fragrance oil (3 drops)

Rosewater Powder (1 tablespoon)

Directions:

Combine all ingredients in a mixing bowl.

Shelf Life: Store for 2 months.

Herb Butter

Ingredients:

Dried mint (2 teaspoon)

Dried sage (2 teaspoon)

Dried rosemary (2 teaspoon)

Cocoa butter (6 ounces)

Crushed organic sea salt (1 cup)

Directions:

Combine all ingredients in a mixing bowl.

Shelf Life: Store for 6 months.

Cucumber Lemon

Ingredients:

Crushed organic sea salt (1/2 cup)

Ripe cucumber (1)

Fresh squeezed lemon juice (2 tablespoon)

Yogurt (2 tablespoon)

Lemon essential oil (2 drops)

Directions:

Chop cucumber into small pieces, add yogurt and lemon then blend to make a paste.

Next, remove from food processor and add salt. Mix thoroughly.

Shelf Life: Store for a week in an air tight container.

Rosemary Peppermint

Ingredients:

Dried rosemary (2 tablespoon)

Crushed organic sea salt (1 cup)

Peppermint fragrance oil (3 drops)

Directions:

Combine all ingredients in a mixing bowl.

Shelf Life: Store for 6 months.

Jasmine and Violet

Ingredients:

Jasmine essential Oil (3 drops)

Violet essential Oil (3 drops)

Crushed organic sea salt (1/2 cup)

Directions:

Combine ingredients in a bowl and mix.

Shelf Life: Store in an air tight container for 6 months.

Hot Buttered Corn

Ingredients:

Crushed organic sea salt (1/2 cup)

Butter (1 teaspoon)

Canola oil (1 teaspoon)

Corn meal (11/4 cup)

Water (11/4 cup)

Directions:

Microwave the cornmeal and water for 1 minute on high temperature.

Combine the remaining ingredients in a mixing bowl.

Leave to cool till room temperature.

Shelf Life: Store in an air tight container for a month.

Autumn Harvest

Ingredients:

Peach fragrance oil (3 drops)

Bergamot Essential Oil (3 drops)

Vanilla Essential Oil (7drops)

Orange fragrance oil (3 drops)

Crushed organic sea salt (1/2 cup)

Directions:

Combine ingredients in a bowl and mix.

Shelf Life: Store for up to 6 months in an air tight container.

Sweet and Salty

Ingredients:

Crushed organic sea salt (1/2 cup)

Organic white sugar (1/2 cup)

Directions:

Combine all ingredients and beat.

Shelf Life: Store for up to 1 week in an air tight container.

Rose Rosemary

Ingredients:

Rose essential oil (3 drops)

Crushed organic sea salt (1/2 cup)

Dried rosemary (2 tablespoon)

Directions:

Combine ingredients and beat with a hand mixer.

Shelf Life: Store in an air tight container for a week.

Apple Pear

Ingredients:

Crushed organic sea salt (1/2 cup)

Small fresh green apple (1)

Small pear (1)

Fresh lemon (2 teaspoons)

Apple fragrance oil (2 drops)

Pear fragrance oil (2 drops)

Directions:

Puree fruit with lemon juice in a blender. Then, combine all ingredients and mix thoroughly.

Shelf Life: Store for a day in an air tight container.

Sweet Potato

Ingredients:

Crushed organic sea salt (1/2 cup)

Cooked sweet potato (1/2 cup)

Ground cinnamon (1 teaspoon)

Directions:

Combine ingredients and beat with a hand mixer.

Shelf Life: Store in an air tight container for to 2 weeks.

Cranberry Almond

Ingredients:

Crushed almonds (1/2 cup)

Crushed organic sea salt (1/2 cup)

Cranberries (2)

Almond oil (2 tablespoon)

Directions:

Combine ingredients in a bowl and mix well.

Shelf Life: Store in an air tight container for 2 months.

Beer And Mayonnaise

Ingredients:

Beer (1/2 cup)

Crushed organic sea salt (1/2 cup)

Mayonnaise (2 tablespoon)

Directions:

Combine all ingredients and beat with a hand mixer.

Shelf Life: Store in an air tight container for 2 weeks.

Pineapple Passion

Ingredients:

Pineapple fragrance oil (3 drops)

Passion fruit fragrance oil (3 drops)

Crushed organic sea salt (1/2 cup)

Fresh pineapple (1/2 cup)

Directions:

Puree fruits in the blender. Mix all ingredients in a bowl and beat with a hand mixer.

Shelf Life: Store in an air tight container for a week.

Egg Protein

Ingredients:

Crushed organic sea salt (1/2 cup)

Large egg (1)

Protein powder (2 tablespoon)

Directions:

Combine ingredients and beat with a hand mixer.

Shelf Life: Store in an air tight container for 2 months.

Strawberry Kiwi

Ingredients:

Strawberry fragrance (3 drops)

Crushed organic sea salt (1/2 cup)

Fresh strawberries (1/4 cup)

Ripe kiwi (1)

Directions:

Combine ingredients and beat with a hand mixer.

Shelf Life: Store for up to 1 week in an air tight container.

OATMEAL BODY SCRUB RECIPES

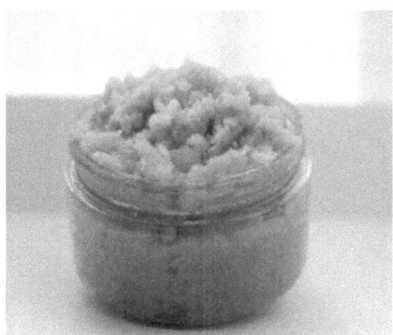

Oats contain grainy substances which have been proven to be very good for facial scrubs. Oats also absorb and remove surface dirt and skin impurities.

Using scrubs made with this wonderful ingredient will help in treating several skin conditions. It works well for dry and itchy skin and is just right for sensitive skin.

Scrubs used with oatmeal will leave your skin soft, silky smooth and hydrated.

Before applying any oatmeal scrub, it is advisable to wash your face with lukewarm water. The scrub can also be used immediately after a shower. This opens up the pores and prepares the skin for improved result.

Grapefruit & Oatmeal Scrub

The use of citrus with oatmeal is a wonderful combination that helps in stimulating, toning and exfoliating the skin.

Ingredients

Fresh Grapefruit (1)

Oatmeal (2 tablespoons)

Directions:

Squeeze juice and pulp out of grapefruit.

Mix with oatmeal till it forms a smooth paste.

Baking Soda & Oatmeal Scrub

The baking soda in this oatmeal scrub serves as a booster. It will soothe your skin in a pleasantly surprising way.

Ingredients

Oatmeal (2 heaping tablespoons)

Baking soda (1 teaspoon)

Directions:

Mix ingredients and add sufficient water to make a sticky paste.

Scrub your face in circular motions, massaging it gently to your skin. Rinse off with lukewarm water.

Oatmeal Sunset Glow

The honey included in this scrub is a natural humectant. It absorbs moisture and keeps it under your skin –just where it ought to be. The apple cider vinegar restores your skin's natural acidity. Vinegar is ideal for both dry and oily complexions as it will keep it softy and fresh.

Ingredients

Oatmeal (8 tablespoons)

Apple cider Vinegar (1 tablespoon)

Dark organic Honey (1 tablespoon)

Finely ground Almonds (2 teaspoon)

Direction:

Put honey in a metal bowl or small glass then warm it in microwave till it becomes runny.

Mix all ingredients until you have a smooth paste

Oatmeal And More

The rich ingredients below is a peek of what to expect –it soothes, exfoliates, cleanse, moisturizes and more!

Ingredients:

Medium Cucumber (1/4 peeled)

Plain unflavored Yogurt (2 tablespoons)

Oatmeal (2 tablespoons)

Jojoba oil   (1 teaspoon)

Sweet Almond oil (1 teaspoon)

Direction:

Slice cucumber and whizz in food processor till it's liquefied.

Add remaining ingredients and mix to make a smooth paste.

Almonds, Avocado & Oatmeal Scrub

Use this avocado based scrub and see how smooth, soft, hydrated and nourished your skin will feel.

Ingredients:

Oatmeal (1 cup)

Coarsely ground Almonds (1 tablespoon)

Peeled ripe Avocado (1)

Direction:

Mix the grounded almonds and oatmeal. Next, mash the peeled avocado to a pulp.

Dip avocado pulp in the almond, oatmeal mix.

Rub and massage on your face very gently, then rinse off.

Cheesy& Juicy Oatmeal Scrub

Cream cheese contains lactic acid that tones and cleanses the skin

Ingredients:

Oatmeal (2 tablespoons)

Cream cheese (1 tablespoon)

Fresh Lemon juice (1 teaspoon)

Direction:

Mix all ingredients until it forms a creamy paste.

Oatmeal &Peels Scrub

A rejuvenating scrub for those who want to smell fresh all day long

Ingredients:

Dried Orange peels (1 cup)

Oatmeal (1 cup)

Finely ground Almonds (2 tablespoon)

Sweet Orange essential oil (1 teaspoon)

Direction:

Put ingredients in a food processor and mix thoroughly. Take a little of this mix in your hand, add some warm water and make a paste. Rub and massage onto your skin.

Cornstarch, Oatmeal And More

A soothing and relaxing body scrub

Ingredients:

Almonds (1/4 cup)

Oatmeal (4 tablespoons)

Cornstarch (1 tablespoon)

Lavender essential oil (2 teaspoons)

Crushed dried Chamomile flowers (1 tablespoon)

Directions:

Place all ingredients in a food processor.

Blend and mash them well.

Take half a tablespoon of this mix in your hand. Add water to make a paste

Cranberries, Coconut Super Oatmeal Scrub

Cranberries have everything your skin needs. Their inclusion in this recipe will help to exfoliate and clean your pores.

The coconut oil is not as greasy as other moisturizers. It is also very effective.

Ingredients

Cranberries (1/2 cup)

Oatmeal (4 tablespoons)

Coconut oil (2 tablespoons)

Sweet Almond oil (1 tablespoon)

Extra virgin Olive oil (1 tablespoon)

Brown Sugar (2 tablespoons)

Directions

Put ingredients in a food processor and mash and blend well.

BOOK 3

100 Plus Essential Oil Healing Recipes

Over 130 Aromatherapy Solutions For Everyday
Ailments, Emotional Health And General Well Being

INTRODUCTION

Essential oils aren't really oils as they do not contain fatty lipids or acids usually found in animal and vegetable oils. They are in fact, highly concentrated volatile oils extracted from aromatic plants and other sources such as barks, roots, flowers and leaves. They are beautifully and uniquely fragrant and give plants their distinctive smells. The fragrant residue of a peeled and squeezed orange, for instance is full of essential oil. Additionally, they vary in colors, evaporate easily into the air, absorb effortlessly into the skin when applied and never go rancid.

Healing Effects of Essential Oils

Essential oils have been used for thousands of years to heal and purify the body of ailments and diseases. Its increase in popularity in this present age may not be unconnected with the accessibility of information on the internet. Additionally, a lot of people are now looking into natural and safe means of maintaining their health and obtaining relief from the very stressful lifestyle that they lead.

Essential oils are an amazing alternative medical treatment. However, they are complimentary and must never be regarded as a substitute to professional medical care. Aromatherapy alone (the use of essential oils for treatments) cannot cure a major illness or permanently cure your stress. What they do is to help in alleviating the symptoms of a physical condition and to temporarily eliminate stress or other psychological factors.

Not everyone responds to essential oil treatment in the same way. This is because essential oils comprise different characteristics so they should be handled differently. 'Stronger or hotter' oils for instance can cause skin irritation for many people. An essential oil that doesn't irritate you can still irritate someone else. Also, if you are allergic to a specific plant, there is a tendency for you to also be allergic to the essential oil where it is extracted from. It is advisable to do a skin test to verify its safeness on your skin.

How to Perform a Skin Patch Test

- Combine 1 drop of essential oil and half a teaspoon of carrier oil (olive or jojoba oil will do). Place 1-2 drops of this combination on the inside of your elbow, wrist or underside of the forearm.
- You may apply a bandage to avoid getting the area wet.
- If you feel any irritation, itching or notice some redness, take away the bandage immediately and wash the area carefully.
- If no irritation happens after a few hours, you can go ahead and use the essential oil in diluted form as it is safe on your skin.

Making& Buying Essential Oils

Essential oils are extracted from plants via distillation and cold pressing (expression). Distillation is the most favorable process of essential oil extraction. It involves heating the plant material by passing steam through it or placing it in water which is then heated.

The heat and steam combination slowly beaks down the plant material and the essential oil is thus released. The essential oil components and steam pass through a pipe to a cooling tank where they go back to liquid form and are collected in a container. The essential oil is then separated from the water and stored.

Expression or cold pressing is used to extract oils that are taken from the rinds of fruits like lime, grapefruit, orange, tangerine and lemon. This method is "cold' because it does not require steam or heat of any kind. Instead, mechanical pressure is literally used to squeeze out the oil from the plant material

The quality of essential oils matter a lot. You need to buy from trusted and reputable source to enjoy effective results. Be wary of mislabeled products. Just because a labeled bottle indicates quality doesn't necessarily mean the content can be trusted.

To test the purity of an essential oil, pour one drop on a clean piece of construction paper. Pure essential oil will evaporate quickly leaving no trace. The presence of a noticeable ring indicates that the oil is diluted.

Diluting Essential Oils With Carrier Oils

Due to essential oils' high concentrative nature, they must be diluted before applying to skin. This can be done effectively with carrier oils.

Carrier oils are pressed from the fatty portions of plants such as the seeds and nuts. As a result, most of them have minimal aroma and minimal color. Some of them also last for a short while as they become rancid after a while. Carrier oils also act as a lubricating agent during massage of larger areas and muscles. They aid absorption as well. Unlike essential oils that evaporate easily when diluted, carrier oils do not.

Ideal carrier oils for essential oils include olive oil, jojoba, sweet almond oil, pomegranate seed oil, pecan oil, evening primrose oil, hemp seed oil, sesame oil, avocado oil, rose hip oil, sunflower oil and many more.

In order to retain the freshness of your carrier oils, keep them from direct light and heat. Make small batches of blends that can be used within a short time. Jojoba oil is very helpful in extending the shelf life of your blend. Essential and carrier oils can also be refrigerated to extend their shelf life.

A 2% dilution is ideal for most aromatherapy applications. Going beyond this measurement may lead to adverse effect. For children and the elderly and individuals with health issues, just 1% dilution of carrier oil is sufficient.

Lavender or melaleuca oils are very mild and can be used undiluted on skin eruptions and burns. Also, the skin of the foot is so thick it is unaffected by undiluted essential oils when applied in that area. However, this does not mean that the essential oil component did not penetrate into the body.

Guidelines For Essential Oils Usage

Essential oils are not supposed to be applied directly on the skin unless appropriately diluted. This is because the potency of these oils can cause an allergic reaction on people with very sensitive skin. Here are some of the most common ways to use essential oils:

Inhalation

Inhalation method is highly effective for emotional and respiratory issues. It could be direct and indirect. Direct inhalation is physically and psychologically beneficial. The aroma stimulates the brain to generate a reaction and when it is inhaled straight into the lungs, the natural constituents can provide therapeutic benefit. However, if you are unsure about your level of sensitivity or reaction to a particular use, do a test with only one drop.

Inhalers: has the advantage of mobility and durability. They are easy to purchase, empty inhalers can also be used as the oil drips easily from the wick.

Tissue cup: Place a few tissue or toilet paper inside a small plastic cup with a lid. Drop 5 drops of oil into it. Open the cup occasionally, hold to the nose and breathe deeply. It can last for about 2 weeks. It is highly stimulating and helpful for staying alert in long meetings and when driving.

Cup and Inhale: helps in stimulating the olfactory cells. The cup and inhale method entails placing a few drops of oil on the palm, cupping the hands over the nose and taking a deep breath. The residue on the hands after an external application can also be used.

Make a spritz: combine 5 –10 drops of oil and half a cup of water. Put the mixture into a spray bottle. Shake well before each use.

Make a steam tent: put some drops of oil into a hot bowl of water. Place a towel over the head, allow it drape around the bowl and then breathe in the vapors. This works really well for colds and sinus problems.

Shirt Tent: Apply the oils to the neck and chest and needed. Put on a T- shirt and while in a relaxed position, pull the neck of the shirt up over the nose and then breathe deeply.

Indirect Inhalation – diffusers

Help to release oils into the air. The body easily absorbs the minute ion particles. They have been proven to improve mental clarity and calm emotions.

Topical Application

Direct - Burns, rashes, cuts, bruise fungal, scrapes bumps, infections and bites are some examples of situations where direct topical application is most effective for pain relief and protection from infection.

Topical administration is also perfect on areas of pain and inflammation such as gout, joint pains, arthritics and muscle aches. Same goes for children who suffer from stomach upset. During application however, caution must be observed to avoid contact of undiluted essential oils with the eyes or mucus membranes.

Compresses: Compresses are helpful after an oil massage. Few drops of essential oil are added to a bowl of hot or cold water. A clean, sterile cotton cloth is dipped into the water and rung out. The cloth is then placed on the affected area until the cloth matches the body temperature. In some cases, oils are used with carrier oil.

Massage : Aromatherapy massage can be administered by massage therapists.

Baths and soakings are another way essential oils can be topically applied. Examples of these are saunas, Jacuzzis, baths and showers.

A full bath aids relaxation: Place oils in water; agitate the water from time to time to eliminate concentration of oils in a particular area and immerse inside it.

Foot bath: There are different types of oils and combination for a range of foot ailments. A few drops released into a bowl of warm water that can contain both feet. Mix well and soak as long as comfortable.

Hand soak: Get a smaller container to fit the hands. Reduce the number of drops of oil to mix well with warm water and soak hands for as long as the solution is comfortable.

Ingestion

While essential oils are used in the food and flavoring industry, internal intake of essential oils should be done with professional advice.

Tea - this is the most common method for ingesting essential oils. 1-2 drops of oil is added to a half cup of warm water and sipped or drunk as needed. Water mustn't be too warm otherwise it will dissipate quickly and the potency will be lost.

Water - Oils are usually added to cold water and ingested e.g. using lemon oil due to its cleansing effect.

Capsules – oils can also be added in a capsule and taken orally like traditional medications. Carrier oil may also be added to the capsule as a buffer to the essential oil.

Swishing - a method of adding 2- 6 drops of oils to a teaspoon of water, swishing in the mouth for 40-60 seconds and swallowing.

Insect Repellent

Many essential oils such as peppermint, lavender and citronella act as a natural repellent against insects. To repel insects, sprinkle some drops of essential oil onto tissues or cotton balls and place them near your doors and windows. Make sure you go through the safety information on the oils you intend to use because some oils may be unsuitable for usage around pets. Also, do not apply the oil directly on fragile surfaces.

Basic Precautions For Essential Oils Usage

- Be careful with sensitive parts of the body like the eyes and ears. On no account should you apply essential oils directly to the ear canal or the eyes. Wash your hand thoroughly after application in order to avoid actions like rubbing the eyes, touching the interior of the nose or handling contact lenses.

- Pregnancy. Although studies have shown that essential oils that are applied topically and after the first trimester cannot harm a developing fetus, it is still advisable to consult a seasoned aromatherapist before usage.

- Some essential oils, mostly citrus oils react to radiant energy, light or other sources of UV rays. Once applied, a rash on the skin or a dark pigmentation shows up within hours or days. It is best to wait for about 6 hours after using any of these photosensitizing oils before exposing the skin to sunlight.

- be careful with babies and individuals with sensitive skin. Some people naturally have sensitive skin so use common sense. Extra caution should be taken when treating babies, small children, and the elderly. This is because they have very sensitive skin that is prone to burning, irritation or stinging sensations. Protect the skin against irritation by using an effective base or carrier oil.

- Keep Out of Reach of Children. Just as you would for medicine, treat essential oils the same way. Essential oils wrongly ingested are harmful and painful as well if accidentally used in the eyes.

- Most essential oils are flammable so keep them from open flame or spark.

-Also, exercise caution with companies that state their product is "Made With Natural Ingredients" or "Made With Essential Oils". Claims like this do not explicitly state that the product is only made with the specified ingredient. It is possible for such products to contain a tiny amount of essential oil just so that they can make the "Made with Essential Oils" claim.

- The lesser the better. Always remember that these oils are highly concentrated so be sure to follow the exact usage. If one drop can deliver the expected results, do not use two.

Blending Essential Oils

Several essential oils can easily be combined to create a blend that can heal, relax and beautify you. This powerful combination is called a synergy blend. Synergy blend oils are a mix of different oils with harmonizing properties. Utilize these oil blends for your medicinal, aromatherapy and cosmetic purposes.

ESSENTIAL OIL RECIPES FOR DIGESTIVE ISSUES

Acid Reflux/Heartburn/Gerd Abdominal Rub

Eucalyptus essential oil - 2 drops

Peppermint essential oil - 1 drop

Fennel essential oil - 2 drops

Grapeseed oil 1 teaspoon (5ml)

Usage:

1. Mix the essential oils with the carrier oil.

2. Rub on the upper abdominal area whenever you have burning pain in your chest.

Acid Reflux/Heartburn/Gerd Drink

Lemon essential oil - 1 drop

Peppermint essential oil - 1 drop

12-16 oz. of drinking water

Usage

1. Add the oil to your water and drink throughout the day.

2. For an intense episode, add 3 drops of Lemon essential oil to a small glass of warm water and drink.

Diarrhea Relief Massage Oil

Lavender essential oil - 2 drops

Peppermint essential oil - 2 drops

Chamomile essential oil - 2 drops

Geranium essential oil - 2 drops

Eucalyptus essential oil - 2 drops

Vegetable carrier oil - 10 ml

Usage:

1. Combine the ingredients in a dark bottle.

2. Rub over abdominal area twice a day.

Diarrhea Capsule Blend

Oregano essential oil - 2 drops

Mountain savory essential oil - 3 drops

Lemon essential oil - 4 drops

Usage:

1. Add 2-3 drops of this blend to 3 drops of vegetable oil in a 00 size capsule and swallow, twice daily.

Diverticulitis Relief Blend

Individuals above the age of forty can develop diverticulitis when there is continuous pressure against weakened tissue. Drinking Aloe Vera juice 2 or 3 times a day can promote healing.

Rosemary essential oil - 2 drops

Peppermint essential oil - 1 drop

Clove essential oil - 1 drop

Chamomile essential oil - 1 drop

Vegetable carrier oil - 1 teaspoon (5ml)

Usage:

1. Blend essential and carrier oils together.

2. Use as massage oil to relieve the discomfort of the ailment.

Indigestion Digestive Stimulant

Roman Chamomile essential oil - 3 drops

Ginger essential oil - 3 drops

Bergamot essential oil - 5 drops

Grapeseed oil - 1 ounce

Usage:

1. Blend the oils in a bottle then use to massage the stomach and the intestinal area rubbing in a clockwise motion.

2. Alternatively, add 1 drop of Lemon or Fennel essential oil to a cup of Chamomile tea and drink.

Motion Sickness Relief

Motion sickness can be relieved and also prevented by the following blend.

Peppermint essential oil - 10 drops

Ginger essential oil - 10 drops

Roman Chamomile essential oil - 10 drops

Usage:

1. Blend all the essential oils in a dark bottle.

2. Put a few drops on a tissue and breathe in. You can also make use of a personal inhaler.

3. Inhale about 30 to 60 minutes before a journey and every 15 to 30 minutes while traveling.

Nausea Instant Remedy

Try this blend whenever you feel queasy.

Lavender essential oil - 1 drop

Peppermint essential oil - 1 drop

Basil essential oil - 1 drop

Carrier oil - 2 teaspoons (10ml)

Usage:

1. Mix the oils with the carrier oil. Massage gently over your abdomen.

2. Before washing your hands, cup your hands over your mouth and nose and inhale slowly a few times.

Abdominal Pain And Cramps Remedy

This blend is effective for abdominal pain that is caused by eating too fast, inflammation of bladder and other digestive problems. Seek medical advice if the pain persists or if there is fever, vomiting, diarrhea or headache.

Calendula essential oil - 1 drop

Clove oil essential oil - 1 drop

Peppermint essential oil - 1 drop

Carrier oil - 1 teaspoon (5 ml)

Usage:

1. Mix together then massage gently on the stomach area using a clockwise motion.

2. Place a warm washcloth on the massaged area for a few minutes to help intensify the effect of the oil blend.

Flatulence (Gas) Relief Capsule

Ginger essential oil

Lavender essential oil

Carrier oil

Usage:

1. Add 1-2 drops of either of these essential oils to 3-4 drops of vegetable oil in an empty size 00, capsule. Take the capsule 15-30 minutes before eating foods that can cause flatulence.

Flatulence (Gas) Massage Blend

This massage blend is recommended when flatulence is accompanied by pain and discomfort.

Peppermint essential oil - 2 drops

Rosemary essential oil - 3 drops

Clove essential oil - 1 drop

Chamomile essential oil - 1 drop

Olive oil - 1 teaspoon (5ml)

Usage:

1. Rub the blend over your abdominal area two times daily.

Bloating Remedy

Lemongrass or Cypress essential oil - 2 drops

Lemon or Grapefruit essential oil - 4 drops

Grapeseed oil - 1 tablespoon

Usage:

1. Blend oils together properly.

2. Massage the swollen area with upward motions, 2 to 3 times daily.

3. Additionally, drink a glass of water to which 1-2 drops of Lemon essential oil has been added 3 times daily.

Constipation Relief Recipe

You are constipated when bowel movements are fewer than 3 to 4 in a week and you should implement this rectifying procedure.

Peppermint essential oil - 5 drops

Lemon essential oil - 10 drops

Rosemary essential oil - 15 drops

Jojoba oil - 30 ml

Usage:

1. Blend oils together then massage in a clockwise motion over the abdominal area three times a day.

ESSENTIAL OIL RECIPES FOR RESPIRATORY PROBLEMS

Bronchitis Relief

Bronchitis occurs when the passage ways in the lungs becomes congested and inflamed, causing breathing difficulty.

Sunflower oil- 1 ounce

Eucalyptus essential oil - 12 drops

Peppermint essential oil - 5 drops

Thyme essential oil - 5 drops

Usage:

Combine ingredients together

Rub gently on your throat and chest several times a day.

Bronchitis Relief For Children

Eucalyptus radiata essential oil - 10 drops

Myrtle essential oil - 25 drops

Thyme linalool essential oil - 10 drops

Niaouli essential oil - 10 drops

Usage

Mix ingredients together.Put 10 drops in a bowl of very hot water and allow the steam to fill the air. Inhaling this steam kills off the germs in the bronchial tubes, trachea and naval cavities. Alternatively, place some drops on a tissue and inhale.

Cold Sores & Fever Blisters Recipe

This blend will enhance healing and reduce the intensity of breakouts.

Roman Chamomile essential oil - 2 drops

Eucalyptus essential oil - 2 drops

Melissa essential oil - 2 drops

Sweet Almond oil - 5 ml

Usage:

1. Mix the ingredients properly.

2. Use a cotton-tip applicator to dab on the blister.

Feet Therapy For Cold & Chilly Feelings

Geranium essential oil - 6 drops

Lemon essential oil - 10 drops

Rosemary essential oil - 4 drops

Usage:

Blend together in an amber bottle.

Add 3-4 drops to a large basin of hot water. (The water mustn't be too hot)

Do not soak feet for more than 30 minutes.

Once done, dry your feet well, apply a little lotion.

Put on your socks, shoes or slipper.

Essential Oil Therapy For Sinusitis

Sinusitis is a very painful condition that is brought about by various causes such as allergies, colds and the flu. When this happens, the protective mucous membranes that is in your sinus cavities become compromised by germs or other irritants, leading to inflammation and infection.

Steaming water -1 quart

Tea tree essential oil - 2 drops

Eucalyptus essential oil - 2 drops

Thyme essential oil - 1 drop

Ginger essential oil - 1 drop

Usage:

Add the essential oils into a 2 quart glass bowl of hot water. (Water mustn't be necessarily steaming).

Hold head over the bowl while draping a towel over head and bowl.

Breathe for 5 to10 minutes. Repeat this up to 6 times every day.

Nasal Inhaler For Chest Congestion

Eucalyptus essential oil - 5 drops

Coarse salt - 1/4 teaspoon

Usage:

Place salt in a small vial with a tight lid. Add essential oil. (The salt absorbs the oil and prevents it from spilling when carried). Open the vial and deeply inhale when needed. Sniff as needed all through the day.

Vapor Rub For Chest Congestion

Eucalyptus essential oil -12 drops

Peppermint essential oil - 5 drops

Thyme essential oil - 5 drops

Olive oil - 1 ounce

Usage:

Combine all ingredients in a glass bottle.

Shake thoroughly to mix evenly.

Massage into chest and throat very gently.

Use one to five times daily and just before bed.

Therapy For Wet Throat Cough

Coughs have distinctive characteristics that can be recognized as either good or bad. The originating cause of a 'bad" cough may be bacterial, viral or symptomatic of another issue entirely.

Peppermint essential oil - 2 drops

Rosemary essential oil - 2 drops

Lime essential oil - 2 drops

Therapy For Deep Painful Chest Cough

Rosemary essential oil - 2 drops

Eucalyptus essential oil - 2 drops

Frankincense essential oil - 2 drops

Therapy For Dry Hacking Cough

Eucalyptus essential oil - 2 drops

Rosemary essential oil - 2 drops

Lemon essential oil- 2 drops

Usage For All Three:

Layer the oils on chest and rub in lightly.

While the oils sits on the skin, cup and inhale deeply from your hands for some minutes.

Next, pull the neck of your shirt over your nose and mouth. Breathe in deeply for some minutes until the aroma starts to dissipate. (Take breaks and then resume if you feel you aren't getting sufficient oxygen).

The oils will penetrate into the lungs and a cooling sensation will be felt.

Do this several times on a daily basis.

Tea Remedy For Cough

Clove and lemon essential oil –1 drop each

Water – 8oz

Honey 1-2 drops (to keep water and essential oils from separating).

 Extra virgin coconut oil carrier (1 tablespoon, optional)

Usage:

Boil water. Add honey and oils to the boiled water. Blend for 60 seconds in a blender at high speed.

Keep a toweled head over the steaming cup to enjoy the therapeutic steam.

Enjoy the great taste as its travels quickly along the esophagus into the body's organs and inner tissues.

EO Gargle Method For Cough

Eucalyptus, Lemon or Peppermint essential oil - 1- 2 drops

Usage:

Put oil(s) in a mouthful (an ounce) of water.

Swallow after gargling.

Breathing Rub for Asthma

Common causes of asthma include stress, allergic reactions to food and airborne allergens. The wheezing characterized of asthma is the result of pushing air through swollen and narrowed bronchial passages. The best time to treat asthma is in-between attacks. Do a sniff test first to ensure there is no adverse reaction.

Jojoba oil - 1 oz

Pine needle essential oil - 3 drops

Eucalyptus essential oil - 3 drops

Tea Tree essential oil - 3 drops

Frankincense essential oil - 2 drops

Thyme essential oil - 2 drops

Myrrh essential oil - 2 drops

Usage:

1. Blend all the oils in a clean PET plastic bottle.

2. Rub on the chest and mid back as often as needed.

Essential Oil Steam for Asthma

Eucalyptus essential oil - 1/4 teaspoon

Water - 3 cups

Usage:

1. Boil water and add essential oils. Drape a towel over the back of the head. Place face over steam and breathe in the steam. Take breaks as needed.

2. Do 3 to 4 rounds of steam inhalation several times every day.

Hay Fever And Other Seasonal Allergies

Eucalyptus essential oil - 4 drops

Chamomile essential oil - 4 drops

Anise essential oil - 3 drops

Lemon essential oil - 3 drops

Petitgrain essential oil - 1 drops

Carrier oil - 5 ml

Usage:

1. Blend the oils properly in a dark bottle.

2. Use 15-20 drops in a bath.

ESSENTIAL OIL RECIPES FOR ACHES & PAINS AROUND THE BODY

Cotton Ball Remedy For Earache

An earache is usually pain in the middle or inner ear. In infants and small children, it is generally the result of irritations brought about by cleaning with a cotton swab or reactions to cleaning products. The trapped fluid puts pressure on the eardrum, causing ache.

Basil essential oil - 3 drops

1/2 of a cotton ball

Grapefruit essential oil - 2 to 3 drops

Usage:

Put the basil on a cotton ball and push it into the ear very lightly. (Do not place the oils directly into the ear as vapor from the cotton ball will get to the infected area).

Leave it overnight.

For additional relief, rub grapefruit oil behind and around the external part of the ear.

Place a warm cloth over the ear, while lying down.

Essential Oil Swab Method

Melrose, lavender or tea-tree essential oil: 2-3 drops

Water

Usage:

Dilute essential oil with warm water.

Swab area around the ear opening, the ear lobe and the exterior part.

Remedy For Mild Tension Headache

A headache is a continuous pain in any region of the head. The brain has pain-sensitive structures and disturbances of these structures causes pain.

Peppermint essential oil – 2-3 drops

Usage:

Rub on the forehead, temples and back of neck.

Remedy For Severe Headache

Apply remedy for mild tension headache.

Compress the aforementioned areas with a clean, damp towel and rest for a few minutes.

Repeat as often as needed. A few drops may be added to the towel to speed up the help.

Keep oils away from eyes.

Migraine Headache Hand Soak

Lavender essential oil - 5 drops

Ginger essential oil - 5 drops

Hot water - 1 quart (about 110°F)

Usage:

Add the essential oils to the hot water.

Soak hands for about 3 minutes.

This therapy may be done repeatedly.

Eyelid Swelling (Sty) Remedy

Lavender or chamomile essential oil

Usage:

Dab with cotton wool 2-3 times daily

EO Topical Remedy For Back Pain

Back pain is a common term that covers a wide range of situations primarily around the spinal column.

Birch, deep blue or wintergreen essential oil – 2- 3 drops

Usage:

Apply topically to the area of pain as often as needed.

Remedy For Back Pain Inflammation Reduction

Black Pepper, basil, wintergreen, bergamot or Rosemary essential oil - 2 to 3drops

Usage:

Apply to spinal area topically.

Oils To Increase Circulation In The Back

Geranium, Citrus Bliss, Eucalyptus, Peppermint, Cypress or Lemon essential oil -2 to3 drops

Usage:

Apply topically to spinal area 2 to 3 times per day

Essential Oils To Eliminate Spasms And Relax Muscles

Chamomile, Marjoram, AromaTouch, Lime or Roman essential oil – 2to3 drops

Usage:

Apply topically to the area where the spasm occurs.

Oils To Heal And Regenerate Tissue

Frankincense, Helichrysum or Sandalwood essential oil: 1 -2 drops

Usage:

Apply twice or thrice daily and topically to the spinal area.

Have a hot compress

EO For Neck Pain Relief

Neck pain usually affects your range of motion. Reduce the spasm and pain in your neck muscles through essential oil application.

Rosemary, peppermint, lavender or juniper essential oil - 5 drops

Usage:

1. Blend the oils in the palm of the hands.

2. Massage mixture into stiff or sore neck.

3. Wrap neck in a scarf for some hours.

Essential Oil Solution For Nose Bleeds

This condition is very common with children. Helichrysum essential oil does not interfere with blood thinning medication.

Helichrysum essential oil- 2- 3 drops

Usage:

1. Apply oil to bleeding nostrils. Apply externally or internally using tissue saturated with helichrysum. The bleeding stops faster with internal application.

Anal Fissures Treatment

These are inflamed tears around the anus caused by straining (usually caused by constipation), excessive rubbing and use of rough toilet paper.

Lavender essential oil - 5 drop

Lemon essential oil - 1 drop

Usage:

1. Add the oils to a bowl of warm water and bathe the area twice daily.

Edema (Swollen Legs, Feet, Ankles, Arms)

This condition occurs as a result of excess fluid in the body tissues at the affected areas. The following blend will strengthen the capillary walls and enhance the drainage of blood.

Cypress essential oil - 3 drops

Lemon essential oil - 5 drops

Grape- seed oil - 1 tablespoon

Usage:

1. Mix oils together and use to massage the affected area. Use upward motions.

2. Repeat 2 to 3 times every day.

ESSENTIAL OIL RECIPES FOR PAINS IN THE BODY

Essential Oil Liniment For Joint Pain

Several factors cause joint pain. They include: injury, overuse and damage from previous injury or disease. The condition may be mild, lasting for a few hours or it may be chronic, lasting for several years. Essential oil helps to limit the inflammation that often comes with it.

Eucalyptus essential oil - 8 drops

Peppermint essential oil - 8 drops

Rosemary essential oil - 8 drops

Cinnamon leaf oil - 4 drops

Juniper berry oil - 4 drops

Marjoram essential oil - 4 drops

Vegetable oil or Alcohol (either rubbing or vodka) - 2 ounces

Usage:

1. Mix ingredients. Stir a few times every day for three days to disperse the oils in the alcohol.

2. This formula must be used only on the painful joints because it is stronger than the typical massage oil so it mustn't be used over a large area of the body. Use several times daily as needed.

Cramp Relief EO For Muscle Pain

Muscles may hurt after a long day of work or vigorous exercise. Repeated daily activities may also tighten muscles, causing them to cramp.

Lavender essential oil - 12 drops

Marjoram essential Oil - 6 drops

Chamomile essential Oil - 4 drops

Ginger essential oil - 4 drops

Vegetable oil - 2 ounces

Usage:

1. Combine all ingredients. Apply daily over the cramping area as often as needed

Nerve Pain Essential Oil Treatment

Damaged nerves can be quite painful because the nerves register pain. Injured nerves also take a long time to regenerate. However, essential oil helps with the treatment process. They relieve pain and speed up healing.

Chamomile essential oil - 4 drops

Marjoram essential oil - 3 drops

Helichrysum oil (optional) - 3 drops

Lavender oil - 2 drops

Vegetable oil - 1 ounce

Usage:

Combine all the ingredients. For pain relief, apply as needed all through the day.

Arthritic Soaking Bath Blend

Bath Salt Blend 1-2 cups

Lavender essential oil - 2 drops

Rosemary essential oil - 2 drops

Juniper berry essential oil - 4 drops

Cypress essential oil - 2 drops

Usage:

Add this blend to bath and soak for 20 to 30 minutes.

Massage Blend For Sore Joints/ Arthritis

Coriander essential oil - 3 drops

Roman Chamomile essential oil - 6 drops

Black Pepper essential oil - 1 drop

Marjoram essential oil - 4 drops

Rosemary essential oil - 3 drops

Ginger essential oil - 1 drop

Carrier Oil of choice - 2 ounces

Usage:

1. Blend well and store in a plastic bottle.

2. Massage daily into sore joints.

Rheumatic Pain Essential Oil Blend

Lavender Essential Oil - 2 drops

Ginger Essential Oil- 4 drops

Silver Fir Essential Oil- 4 drops

Carrier oil of choice- 4 teaspoons

Usage:

Combine and apply on affected areas.

Achy Muscle Soother

Lemongrass essential oil – 2 drops

Ginger essential oil - 4 drops

Lavender essential oil - 4 drops

Almond oil - 4 teaspoons

Usage:

Combine and apply on affected areas.

Tendonitis Relief With Essential Oil

Tendonitis is simply the inflammation of a tendon. While overuse is the main cause of this often painful and debilitating condition, it can also be brought about by infection or rheumatic disease. Knee, ankle, wrist or Achilles tendonitis along with the elbow, foot and wrist pain that comes with them are difficult to treat. However, natural essentials oils can offer a measure of relief and quicken the healing process.

Basil essential oil -10 drops

Wintergreen essential oil - 8 drops

Cypress essential oil - 6 drops

Peppermint essential oil - 3 drops

Usage:

1. Mix oils together, rub on location. Can also be mixed with 2 tbsp of jojoba oil and massage larger areas of the body.

ESSENTIAL OIL RECIPES FOR SKIN BLEMISHES/COSMETIC PROBLEMS

Aromatherapy Treatment For Acne

It's ok to have one or two pimples now and then but when breakouts are frequent; this blend can be very helpful.

Geranium essential oil - 3 drops

Tea Tree or Lemongrass essential oil - 7 drops

Lavender essential oil - 10 drops

Jojoba oil or Aloe Vera gel - 30ml

Usage:

1. Mix jojoba oil with essential oils in a dark glass bottle.

2. Apply a little quantity to affected areas of the skin twice a day. Avoid eyes, lips and nose.

3. Results will appear if used consistently for a few weeks.

Relief For Prickly Heat Rash In Children

Use this combination for babies two years and under. Older children will require double the measurement.

Lavender essential oil - 2 drops

Baking Soda - 1/4 cup

Usage:

1. Mix the two ingredients together then add to bath water.

Itchy Skin Recipe

Lavender essential oil - 5 drops

Tea Tree essential oil - 3 drops

Frankincense essential oil - 2 drops

Witch hazel - 2 ounces

<u>**Usage:**</u>

1. Fill a 2 ounce spray bottle halfway with witch hazel, add the essential oils, shake together then fill remaining space with witch hazel.

2. Apply this mixture on itchy skin.

Remedy For Liver Spots (Age Spots)

Frankincense essential oil - 2 drops

Lavender essential oil - 2 drops

Myrrh essential oil - 2 drops

Extra virgin coconut oil - 10ml

<u>**Usage:**</u>

1. Mix the ingredients together and apply topical at least once a day.

Dark circles Or Bags Under Eyes

Roman Chamomile essential oil - 1 drop

Lavender essential oil - 1 drop

Aloe Vera gel or other lotion/cream - 30mls

Usage:

1. Mix the essential oils properly with aloe vera gel.

2. Once a day, cleanse and dry the face then rub the blend very gently below and above the eye socket.

3. Avoid contact with eyelids or eyelashes so you will not get some in your eyes.

Healing Blend For Chapped Lips

Geranium essential oil - 2 drops

Chamomile essential oil - 1 drop

Rose essential oil - 2 drops

Neroli essential oil - 1 drop

Aloe Vera oil - 20 ml

Usage:

1. Mix and apply this blend to chapped lips for healing and pain relief.

Treatment For Cracked Skin

The Lavender oil in this blend will help to fight infected cracks in the skin. You should also endeavor to drink adequate water daily to keep your body hydrated.

Lavender essential oil - 10 drops

Helichrysum essential oil - 5 drops

Neroli essential oil - 5 drops

Lotion - 1 ounce

Usage:

1. Mix the essential oils with 1 ounce of your body lotion and apply as many times as necessary daily. It will stimulate healing of cracks and the regeneration of new cells.

Dry Skin Moisturizer

Geranium essential oil - 7 drops

Sandalwood essential oil - 10 drops

Rosewood essential oil - 3 drops

Ylang Ylang essential oil - 5 drops

Carrier oil - 2 ounces

Usage:

1. Mix all ingredients together in a bottle.

2. Apply 4 - 6 drops of this blend to dry area twice a day.

Oily Skin Remedy

Geranium essential oil - 3 drops

Grapefruit essential oil - 3 drops

Lavender essential oil - 3 drops

Evening primrose carrier oil - 30ml

Usage:

1. Mix the ingredients in a glass bottle and apply a little quantity to your face every day.

Oily Skin And Acne Steam Bath

This recipe is good for stimulating facial skin.

Lemon essential oil - 4 drops

Juniper Berry essential oil - 6 drops

Cypress essential oil - 4 drops

Usage:

1. Add the oils above to a bowl of hot water.

2. Bend over the bowl; drape a towel over your head and the bowl to prevent the escape of steam.

3. Hold this position for 5-10 minutes then use tepid water to rinse your face and pat dry.

Skin Firming Remedy For Flabby Skin

If your skin is sagging after weight loss, the usage of aromatherapy oils can restore elasticity and improve blood flow.

Patchouli essential oil - 8 drops

Cypress essential oil - 5 drops

Geranium essential oil - 5 drops

Sandalwood essential oil - 1 drop

Jojoba oil - 1/2 teaspoon

Usage:

1. Mix these ingredients together to make a soothing skin serum.

2. Massage affected areas before bed at night and sometimes in the morning.

Stretch Marks Treatment Lotion

Lavender essential oil - 3 drops

Frankincense essential oil - 3 drops

Geranium essential oil - 3 drops

Helichrysum essential oil - 3 drops

Virgin coconut oil - 1 ounce

Usage:

1. Use this blend as body lotion on affected areas.

Stretch Marks Cocoa Butter Cream

Neroli essential oil - 4 drops

Cocoa butter (deodorized) - 3 ounces

Avocado oil - 1 ounce

Usage:

1. Melt cocoa butter in a double boiler then stir in avocado oil.

2. Pour the mixture in a bowl to cool then add the essential oil.

3. Transfer to a 4 ounce jar with a lid and use as body cream.

4. Store in the refrigerator to avoid the growth of mold.

Wrinkles And Mature Skin Blend

Frankincense - 5 drops

Lavender - 15 drops

Carrot seed - 5 drops

Neroli - 5 drops

Jojoba oil - 2 ounces

Usage:

1. Mix ingredients together in a dark bottle.

2. Massage the affected areas as needed.

Sun Spots Aromatherapy Remedy

Frankincense essential oil - 5 drops

Lavender essential oil - 5 drops

Distilled water

Usage:

1. Mix these essential oils with water in a 2 ounce spray bottle.

2. Spray this mixture on your skin before rubbing on your sunscreen or moisturizer every other day.

Sunburn Spray Soother

Lavender oil - 20 drops

Aloe Vera juice - 4 ounces

200 IU vitamin E oil

Vinegar - 1 tablespoon

Usage:

1. Combine all the ingredients. Place in a spritzer bottle. Shake well before using as often as needed.

2. Keeping the spray refrigerated provides extra relief due to the coolness.

Sunscreen Recipe

Helichrysum essential oil - 30 drops

Lavender essential oil - 30 drops

Fractionated Coconut oil

Usage:

1. Add the essential oils to 2 ounce spray bottle then fill up the bottle with fractionated coconut oil.

2. Shake and spray on your body as sunscreen.

Aromatherapy For Scars

Scars can develop from scrapes, cuts or surgery. You can reduce the visibility of these blemishes with the use of essential oils.

Helichrysum essential oil - 6 drops

Lavender essential oil - 4 drops

Rosehip seed oil - 1 ounce

Usage:

1. Mix this combination in a bottle.

2. Start using daily on the cut once it is sealed shut (this could be after a few days). Apply the blend over the scab and the immediate area. Do not remove the scabs on the surface. Picking or removing scabs will lead to scarring.

3. If you had a surgery, start applying the blend once the staples and sutures are removed.

4. This blend can also be used on old scars but it takes 3-6 months to get results.

ESSENTIAL OIL RECIPES HAIR CARE

Remedy For Light Dandruff

Dandruff occurs when excessive skin oils and cells die and flake off in unusually large quantities. Although not a serious condition, it is often embarrassing.

Melaleuca -2 to 3 drops

Any high quality shampoo

Usage

Add oil to shampoo and use.

Essential Oil Blend For Heavy Dandruff

Any carrier oil - 1 teaspoon

Lemon essential oil - 4 drops

Lavender essential oil - 4 drops

Melaleuca essential oil- 4 drops

Rosemary essential oil- 4 drops

Usage

Massage blend into the scalp every night. Cover with shower cap. Shampoo it out the following morning.

Essential Oil To Prevent Flaking From Harsh Hair Products

Break the cycle of damaged scalp and flaking caused by substandard dandruff shampoos by using the following:

Birch, Wintergreen or Rosemary - 4 -6 drops

Shampoo - 1/2 ounce

Usage

1. Mix oil into shampoo. Apply1 inch partings in the hair and then rub mixture into scalp.

2. Leave on for 5-7 minutes and then apply regular shampoo and conditioning.

Mild Hair Loss Remedy

Mix together 1 - 2 drops of Rosemary essential oil to shampoo

Use it every day to stimulate follicle

Serious Hair Loss Remedy

Rosemary essential oil - 3 drops

Lavender essential oil - 5 drops

Cypress essential oil - 4 drops

Clary Sage essential oil - 4 drops

Sandalwood - 10 drops

Usage:

Combine all ingredients and pour in your hair shampoo.

ESSENTIAL OIL RECIPES FOR SKIN PROBLEMS

Aromatherapy Treatment Of Boils

Boils can appear on different parts of the body and can sometimes be associated with fever and fatigue.

Tea tree essential oil - 2 drops

Lavender essential oil - 2 drops

Juniper essential oil - 1 drop

Usage:

1. Dilute the essential oils in 200 ml of hot water.

2. Bathe the infected area twice daily with this mixture.

3. 1drop of Chamomile essential oil should be added if there is severe inflammation.

Ringworm Treatment

The Melaleuca and Thyme in this blend are effective against fungal infections while the Lavender will aid healing of the skin.

Melaleuca essential oil - 30 drops

Thyme essential oil - 30 drops

Lavender essential oil - 30 drops

Usage:

1. Apply 2-3 drops of this combination topically on infected area 3 times daily for 10 to 12 days

Scabies Aromatherapy Treatment

Peppermint essential oil - 4 drops

Lavender essential oil - 4 drops

Sweet Almond oil - 1 teaspoon

Usage:

1. Apply this blend to itching areas 2-3 times a day, after a bath.

2. Wash clothing of affected person at high temperature. Spray pillows, mattresses, couches with a mixture of 5% lavender, 5% white camphor and 90% alcohol. Wear a mask while spraying to avoid inhaling.

Eczema And Dermatitis Treatment

This blend will relieve itching, sooth the skin and also stimulate healing.

Helichrysum essential oil - 5 drops

Melaleuca essential oil- 3 drops

Lavender essential oil - 10 drops

Myrrh essential oil - 5 drops

Extra virgin coconut oil - 1 teaspoon

Usage:

1. Mix together and apply topically on affected area daily.

Remedy For Warts

Lemon essential oil - 12 drops

Bergamot FCF essential oil - 4 drops

Tea Tree essential oil - 4 drops

Cypress essential oil - 3 drops

Thyme essential oil - 4 drops

Jojoba oil - 1 tablespoon

Usage:

1. Blend together in a dark glass bottle.

2. Apply 2 drops of this blend to the wart then cover with a Band-Aid.

3. Do this once a day for 2 weeks.

Note: Use 2 teaspoons of jojoba oil if using on the elderly or children.

Shingles Relief With Essential Oil

Shingles is a skin rash caused by an inflammation of the nerve and skin. It is caused by the same virus that causes chicken-pot.

Melaleuca essential oil - 30 drops

Eucalyptus essential oil - 30 drops

Lavender essential oil - 30 drops

Usage:

1. Mix and add to a 4-ounce spray bottle. Fill it with fractionated coconut oil. Shake thoroughly before spraying.

2. Spray directly to affected area as often as needed to deal with the pain.

Bed Sores (Pressure Ulcers)

Bedsores or pressure ulcers are injuries that often develop from continuous pressure applied to the skin when in a limited area. People who are confined to a chair or bed for an extended period usually experience this problem.

Lavender essential oil- 10 drops

Helichrysum essential oil -6 drops

Myrrh essential oil -6 drops

Geranium essential oil -4 drops

Melaleuca essential oil -4 drops

2 tbs. FCO or EVCO carrier oil

Usage:

Apply topically thrice a day

Emergency Burn Wash/Compress

While Second and third degree burns call for immediate medical attention, first degree burns as well as sunburns can be subdued by essential oils. Essential oils also provide protection from bacterial infection that usually occurs with burns.

Lavender oil- 5 drops

Water - 1 pint, about 50°F

Usage:

1. Add essential oil to water, stirring thoroughly to disperse the oil.

2. Dip the burned area in the water for a few minutes. Alternatively, soak a soft cloth in the water and apply to burned area. Leave the compress on for 15-20 minutes then soak again and reapply 2-3 times more.

ESSENTIAL OIL RECIPES FOR INSECT AND ANIMAL BITES

Essential Oil For Gnat And Chigger Bites

Although bites and stings from insects such as mosquitoes and ants produce a lot of discomfort, including redness and swelling, they can easily be dealt with. However, bites from insects like scorpions and black widow are usually very harmful and must seriously be attended to. In both cases, essential oil can provide a measure of relief.

Cider vinegar - 1 teaspoon

Thyme essential oil - 3 drops

Usage:

Clean bitten area with warm soapy water, rinse and dry.

Combine the oil and vinegar and dab on affected area for relief.

Mosquito And Other Minor Insect Bites

Lavender, peppermint or tea tree essential oil - 1-3 drops

Usage:

For relief from itching, dab oil topically on affected area.

Repeat every 1-2 hours if necessary.

For very sensitive skin and for young children, dilute essential oil with a carrier oil

Note: Chamomile essential oils can reduce swelling and inflammation

Remedy For Bee Stings And Serious Insect Bites

Remove the stinger first.

Then apply lavender or roman chamomile as above.

Apply a cold compress over bitten area, changing regularly.

Do NOT use ice as it could cause damage the skin if it becomes accidentally frozen.

Seek immediate medical assistance if allergic to bee stings or others.

Essential Oil To Repel Bugs

Lemon essential oil - 19 drops

Cajeput essential oil - 25 drops

Cedarwood essential oil - 13 drops

Geranium essential oil - 19 drops

Sweet almond oil - 2 oz

Usage:

Mix all the essential oils in a recyclable Plastic bottle.

Add the almond oil and Shake until thoroughly blended.

Apply thinly to exposed skin as needed.

Dog Bite Relief Blend

If there is no broken skin, clean the area and apply 1-2 drops of Melaleuca topically.

1. for puncture wound:

- Clean the area and apply 1 to 2 drops of Frankincense topically.

-Dilute with carrier oil so the oils can penetrate easily into the puncture.

 - Bandage and treat twice per day for 2 to 3 days.

2. for open wounds with torn flesh:

-Stop the bleeding using Helichrysum and pressure.

-Clean the area and then topically apply melaleuca and frankincense.

3. Note: If skin is damaged to the point where stitches are required or there is danger of damaged bones, tendons, ligaments or nerves, seek immediate professional medical assistance. Additionally, if there is risk of rabies, the animal should be captured if possible.

ESSENTIAL OIL RECIPES FOR ORAL HEALTH

EO Simple Mouth Wash

Peppermint essential oil - 2 drops

Lemon essential oil - 4 drops

Distilled water- 2 cups

Usage:

1. Add oils to water. Shake thoroughly before each use.

2. Swish a mouthful for 1 to 2 minutes and spit out.

Gum Essential Oil Blend

Tea Tree essential oil - 10 drops

Peppermint essential oil - 1 drop

Lemon essential oil - 3 drops

Myrrh essential oil - 6 drops

Almond oil - 1 teaspoon

Usage:

1. After brushing the teeth and rinsing the mouth with mouthwash, combine the above oils and apply a small quantity on your gums daily.

2. Consult your dentist if the gums or the source of irritation do not heal.

Therapeutic Fresh Breath Mouthwash

Tea Tree essential oil - 2 drops

Myrrh essential oil - 2 drops

Peppermint essential oil - 1 drop

Distilled water - 4 to 8 Ounces

Usage:

1. Mix together in a glass or plastic PET bottle. Shake well before use.

2. Swish about 1/2 ounce in your mouth after eating as required or after brushing your teeth.

Neck Wrap Remedy For Sore Throat

Sore throat may be caused by bacterial infection, yelling, lots of talking or singing. Sometimes, the throat may be so inflamed that swallowing will be difficult.

Lavender essential oil - 2 drops

Bergamot essential oil - 2 drops

Tea tree essential oil - 1 drop

Hot water - 2 cups

Usage:

1. Mix essential oils with water. Soak a flannel in the still warm water, wring it out.

2. Wrap around neck and then cover with a thin towel to retain the heat. Take it off before it becomes cold. Use all through the day as frequently as you desire.

Throat Gargle/Spray For Sore Throat

Marjoram essential oil - 4 drops

Warm water - 1/2 cup

Salt - 1/2 teaspoon

Usage:

1. Combine the ingredients.

2. Shake thoroughly to disperse the oils and dissolve the salt before spraying or gargling.

3. Gargle every 30 minutes initially and then several times daily.

Toothache Oil Blend

Clove bud essential oil - 4 drops

Orange essential oil (for flavor) - 1 drop

Vegetable oil - 1 teaspoon

Usage:

1. Combine ingredients and then rub a few drops onto the painful gums. Repeat frequently.

2. Put clove bud in the most painful area of the mouth during an emergency. Gently mash the clove with the teeth as it softens. This way, the oil is released and you can then suck on it.

3. Some young children may find clove oil too hot for them. You can replace it with chamomile oil. Since chamomile is less effective as a pain killer, apply treatment as frequently as possible.

Tonsillitis Essential Oil Relief

Tonsillitis simply means inflammation of the tonsils. It is generally caused by viral or bacterial infection. It may be treated via different medical procedures but essential oil basically helps to lessen the swelling and discomfort.

Water - 1 qt

Lemon, lavender or eucalyptus essential oil - 3 drops

Usage:

1. Boil water and add the essential oils. Place toweled head over hot pot of water. Breathe the aroma.

2. May also be drank as tea to relieve sore throat or used in a warm bath.

Bad Breath Due To Digestive Issues

Peppermint essential oil - 2 drops

Lemon essential oil - 2 drops

Brandy - a teaspoon

Bad Breath Due To Gum Disease

Tea tree essential oil - 2 drops

Thyme essential oil - 2 drops

Usage For Both Recipes

1. Dilute the essential oil in brandy. Add mixture to a glass of warm water.

2. Sip, swirl around then mouth and spit out. Do not swallow.

Remedy For Mouth Ulcers (Stomatitis)

Mouth ulcers also called stomatitis or canker sores mostly occur on the tongue, inner lip, inner cheek, floor of the mouth and soft palate. The condition is usually painful, making it difficult to eat and chew. It is caused by a variety of factors including dietary deficiencies, Candida and friction from a denture.

Myrrh essential oil - 3 drops

Alcohol - 1 teaspoon

Usage:

1. Using a cotton-bud, dab directly onto the ulcer. (May sting for a while but is often very effective).

2. Alternatively, dilute with half a glass of water and make into a mouthwash.

Mouth Alcer Treatment For Children

Myrrh essential oil is extremely bitter especially for children so it is best to add Peppermint, mandarin or Fennel oil to this mixture.

Myrrh essential oil - 2 drops

Peppermint essential oil - 1 drop

Alcohol - 1 teaspoon

Usage:

1. Using a cotton-bud, dab directly onto the ulcer.

2. Alternatively, dilute with half a glass of water and make into a mouthwash.

ESSENTIAL OIL RECIPES FOR FOOT AND LEG CARE

Simple Foot Powder Blend

Thyme essential oil - 2 drops

Tea Tree essential oil - 2 drops

Rosemary essential oil - 5 drops

Talc Powder - 5 oz

Usage:

1. Place oils in powder. Shake thoroughly and let it sit for 24 hours. Before using on your feet, shake again. Use daily.

2. Dust on your feet after showering. Be sure to spread your toes.

Food Bath Blend (for tired feet)

Grapefruit essential oil - 4 drops

Myrtle essential oil - 4 drops

Cajeput essential oil - 3 drops

Spearmint essential oil - 4 drops

Sesame, Almond or Hazelnut carrier oil -1 teaspoon

Usage:

1. Blend all ingredients and add to a basin of warm water. Swirl around and then soak in your feet.

2. Relax for about 15 minutes.

Essential Oil Preparation For Dry Cracked Heels

Geranium essential oil - 10 drops

Melaleuca essential oil- 10 drops

Peppermint essential oil -10 drops

Virgin Coconut Oils - 1 tablespoon

Usage:

1. Blend together. Apply topically on area every morning and evening.

2. Cover with socks

Essential Oil Blend For Calluses And Corns

Although calluses are generally painless, they tend to be painful on the bottom of feet where they occur due to poorly fitting shoes. Corns occur above the toe joints and they can cause a lot of discomfort as well.

Myrrh essential oil - 6 drops

Vanilla essential oil - 4 drops

Lavender essential oil - 12 drops

Sweet almond - 2 ounces

Usage:

1. Mix together in a bottle, shaking well to mix.

2. Massage into the affected area to soften calluses and corns. Apply daily.

Remedy For Foot Odor

Lavender- 2-3 drops

Basin of lukewarm water

Usage:

1. Add oil to bath and then place feet (safe for blistered and cracked feet as well) in it for 10- 15 minutes.

Anti-Fungus Blend For Athletic Foot

Sweaty feet that are cloistered in socks and shoes are the leading cause of Athlete's foot. Such moist environments attract fungus.

Tea tree essential oil - 12 drops

Geranium essential oil   8 drops

Thyme essential oil - 3 drops

Tincture of benzoin - 1 tablespoon

Apple cider vinegar - 2 ounces

Myrrh essential oil - 2 drops (optional)

Usage:

1. Combine all ingredients. Shake well before use.

2. Use as wash daily or as often as needed or dab on afflicted area.

Athletic Foot Fungal Powder

Lemon eucalyptus or tea tree essential oil - 14 drops

Geranium essential oil - 8 drops

Sage essential oil - 5 drops

Peppermint essential oil - 1 drop

Cornstarch - 1/4 cup

Usage:

1. Place the cornstarch in a plastic bag. Gently sprinkle in the essential oils, evenly distributing them through the powder.

2. Next, close the bag and then toss the powder. This will break up any formed clumps. Store the powder in a glass or ceramic container or a sealed plastic bag. A perforated lidded shake bottle will even make dispensing easier to achieve. Use powder once daily or as often as needed.

Gout Relief Blend

This blend is effective for the common gout that comes with intense pain and redness of the big toe.

Frankincense essential oil 10 drops

Basil essential oil - 10 drops

Usage:

1. Mix the oils together in a dark bottle.

2. Apply 2-3 drops of the blend to the painful area then cover with hot compress.

3. Repeat 2 or 3 times per day.

ESSENTIAL OIL RECIPES FOR CUTS, BRUISES & BONES

Balm Relief For Minor Cuts And Scrapes

Minor cuts are scrapes are inevitable. This balm recipe prepares you for immediate aromatherapy treatment when one is needed.

Lavender essential oil - 40 drops

Tea Tree essential oil - 40 drops

Grated Beeswax - 1 ounce

Vegetable carrier oil (Jojoba, Sweet Almond Oil) - 3 ounces

Wide-mouth jar - 4 ounce

Usage:

1. In a double boiler, heat the beeswax at low setting. In a separate pan, slowly heat your carrier oil. Next, pour the heated carrier into a medium bowl. Add the melted beeswax, stirring thoroughly.

2. Add lavender and tea tree essential oils, stirring well again. Pour this mixture into a wide-mouth jar. Leave to cool for about 5-10 minutes before tightening with the lid. Wait until cooled before using.

3. To use: clean the minor cuts and scrapes and then apply a thin amount of the balm. Bandage if necessary

Essential Oil Blend For Bruises

As anti-inflammatory oil, helichrysum essential oil is remarkable and helps to ease the discomfort and unsightliness of bruising.

Helichrysum essential oil - 8 drops

Jojoba or sweet almond oil- 1 ounce

Usage:

1. Combine both oils, mixing well.

2. Store in a dark colored glass bottle.

Germ Fighter Spray (to prevent infection and foster healing)

Tea tree essential oil -12 drops

Eucalyptus essential oil - 6 drops

Lemon essential oil - 6 drops

Distilled water - 2 ounces

Usage:

Combine ingredients. Dispense formula from a spray bottle. Before each use, shake well to disperse the oils.

Pain Relief Blend (To calm the wounded)

Lavender essential –2 or 3 drops

Usage:

Apply directly to wound. Put also on the palms, rub together and inhale the oil's calming fragrance.

Essential Oil Blend For Bone Spurs

Bone spurs (osteophytes) is simply an added bone growth to a normal bone area. This condition usually occurs after an injury as the body attempts to repair itself. Common activities like running, dancing and even wearing tight shoes can cause bone spurs.

Wintergreen essential oil - 4 drops

Eucalyptus essential oil - 4 drops

Marjoram essential oil - 4 drops

Cypress essential oil - 4 drops

Helichrysum essential oil - 4 drops

Peppermint essential oil - 4 drops

Frankincense essential oil - 4 drops

Coconut oil carrier - 10 drops

Usage:

1. Mix ingredients and apply to affected area twice daily until the bone spur gone.

2. Continue for more 2 weeks. Wrap with a warm cloth to speed up results and then wrap with plastic bag and extra towel to keep heat in.

Alternative Bone Spur Solution

Eucalyptus essential oil - 5 drops

Marjoram essential oil - 5 drops

Cypress essential oil - 5 drops

Lavender essential oil - 5 drops

Thyme essential oil - 5 drops

Basil essential oil - 5 drops

Coconut carrier oil - 30 drops

Usage:

1. Mix ingredients and apply to affected area twice daily until the bone spur gone.

2. Continue for more 2 weeks. Wrap with a warm cloth to speed up results and then wrap with plastic bag and extra towel to keep heat in. Reported results took between 2 weeks to 3 months.

Remedy For Broken Bones

Broken or fractured bones can happen anywhere in the body. Here are the essential oils that will help:

- For pain relief: Wintergreen essential oil

- For healing: Birch essential oil (bone repair), Helichrysum (nerve damage, overall tissue regeneration and repair), Cypress (circulation), Lemongrass essential oil (ligaments), White Fir (anti-inflammatory) and Marjoram (tissue rebuilding).

- For stress relief: Lavender essential oil

<u>Usage:</u>

1. Apply 1-2 drops topically to injured area 2- 3 times daily.

ESSENTIAL OIL RECIPES FOR EMOTIONAL HEALTH

Alertness And Energizing Blend

Use this blend when you have demanding tasks ahead of you and you want to be mentally alert and aware.

Juniper essential oil - 14 drops

Rosemary essential oil - 8 drops

Pine needle essential oil - 8 drops

Usage:

1. Blend all the ingredients in a dark bottle.

2. Place several drops in your home, office or car diffuser (for long distance driving).

3. When diffusing in the car, use only for 20 minutes at a time.

Anxiety Relief Recipe

It is not always possible to avoid things that make you anxious. You can however handle uncertainties better when you use nerve-calming essential oils.

Geranium essential oil - 2 drops

Vanilla essential oil - 2 drops

Neroli essential oil - 3 drops

Rosewood essential oil - 2 drops

Frankincense essential oil - 1 drop

Ylang ylang essential oil - 2 drops

Rose essential oil - 1 drop

Usage:

1. Mix properly in dark glass bottle.

2. Use in a nasal inhaler or just place 1-2 drops on tissue or cotton ball and inhale.

Romantic Massage Blend

Several essential oils can enhance the feeling of excitement and stimulate sensations *for romantic encounters.*

Orange essential oil - 2 drops

Jasmine essential oil - 2 drops

Ylang ylang essential oil - 1 drop

Sandalwood essential oil - 2 drops

Almond oil - 1 ounce

Usage:

1. Mix the ingredients properly.

2. Use for a slow and loving, romantic massage.

Aphrodisiac For Love And Romance

Sandalwood essential oil - 3 drops

Rose essential oil - 2 drops

Lotion - 1 or 2 tablespoons

Usage:

1. Mix the essential oils into 1 or 2 tablespoons of your body lotion.

2. Apply on your arms, face and body.

Aromatherapy For Burnout, Exhaustion And Fatigue

These oils can rejuvenate and lift you up when you have been through a physically and mentally exhaustive circumstance.

Lime essential oil - 15 drops

Grapefruit essential oil - 8 drops

Cardamom essential oil - 8 drop

Usage:

1. Add a few drops into a diffuser in the room where you are resting.

2. Mix with 2 ounces of almond oil and treat yourself to a relaxing massage to release tense muscles.

Note: Exhaustion and burnout will require several days of adequate rest and sleep.

Seasonal Affective Disorder (SAD) And Cabin Fever

It is natural for some people to have the blues for one or two days when the seasons are changing.

Geranium essential oil - 15 drops

Bergamot essential oil - 10 drops

Lavender essential oil - 5 drops

Usage:

1. Blend the oils together and use in a diffuser.

2. Add 6-8 drops of this blend to the bath tub and soak in the water.

Note: Endeavor to go outside within the daylight hours to make you feel better during this time.

Concentration Enhancing Blend

Lemon essential oil - 20 drops

Basil essential oil - 6 drops

Rosemary essential oil - 2 drops

Usage:

1. Mix these essential oils together then diffuse into the air.

2. If you are at work, you can place a personal diffuser on your desk or just put a few drops of the blend on tissue for inhaling.

Confidence Booster

When you feel confident, it is easier to tackle tasks and challenges more effectively. This blend will give you the needed emotional support to strengthen your confidence.

Orange essential oil - 10 drops

Grapefruit essential oil - 10 drops

Bergamot essential oil - 5 drops

Usage:

1. Mix the oils together and use several drops in an inhaler.

Confidence Boosting Rub

Rosemary essential oil - 20 drops

Fennel essential oil - 10 drops

Carrier oil or lotion - 2 ounces

Usage:

1. Mix together the ingredients and apply to your skin when needed.

Happiness Enhancing Blend

Although essential oils cannot create happiness, they can help to clear your mind so you can focus on things that make you happy. Use the following blend to bring up your spirits.

Rose geranium essential oil - 5 drops

Orange essential oil - 19 drops

Cinnamon essential oil - 1 drop

Clove essential oil - 1 drop

Usage:

1. Blend these oils and use in a diffuser.

2. Use 5 drops in your bath.

Comfort For Grief and Loss

It is natural to go through a period of grief when you lose a loved one, a job or a pet. Essential oils can help with the sorrow and sadness being experienced at this time.

Vanilla essential oil - 5 drops

Mandarin essential oil - 3 drops

Rose Otto essential oil - 3 drops

Roman Chamomile essential oil - 3 drops

Usage:

1. Blend the oils in a dark glass bottle and use in your diffuser.

2. Blend oils with 1 ounce of Almond or Jojoba oil and use for massage.

Insomnia Sleep Time Blend

In addition to using this blend, you should also avoid stimulating foods like coffee, colas and some teas in the evening and also avoid stimulating entertainment (movies or talk shows) close to bedtime.

Sandalwood essential oil - 6 drops

Ylang Ylang essential oil - 2 drops

Neroli essential oil - 2 drops

Vetiver essential oil - 1 drop

Coriander essential oil - 1 drop

Jojoba oil - 1 tablespoon

Usage:

1. Blend essential oils with Jojoba.

2. Take a warm bath before bedtime then apply this blend to pulse points such as inside of the wrists, behind the ears and behind the knees.

Insomnia Massage Blend

Marjoram essential oil - 1 drop

Ylang Ylang essential oil - 1 drop

Roman Chamomile essential oil - 1 drop

Sweet Orange essential oil - 1 drop

Tangerine essential oil - 1 drop

Lavender essential oil - 1 drop

Carrier oil - 1 ounce

Usage:

1. Mix the oils together and massage your body at bedtime.

Memory Loss Recovery Blend

Memory loss is predominant in the elderly but it can also be experienced occasionally by younger people. Essential oils like Rosemary and Basil are used for dementia and Alzheimer's patients in many nursing facilities.

Basil essential oil - 6 drops

Lemon essential oil - 20 drops

Rosemary essential oil - 2 drops

Usage:

1. Mix the oils together and use in a diffuser.

Nervousness And Anxiety

Here is a useful anti-anxiety blend.

Lavender essential oil - 10 drops

Orange essential oil -10 drops

Marjoram essential oil - 2 drops

Cedarwood essential oil - 2 drops

Sweet Almond oil - 4 ounces

Usage:

1. Combine ingredients in a small glass bottle.

2. Open and inhale whenever you feel nervous.

Stress Eliminating Recipe

Lavender essential oil - 15 drops

Lemon essential oil - 10 drops

Clary Sage essential oil - 5 drops

Usage:

1. Mix together in an amber bottle.

2. Use in a diffuser or personal nasal inhaler.

3. Add 5-6 drops of this blend to warm bath water and soak in it for 20-30 minutes.

Positive Energy Recipe

Orange essential oil - 4 drops

Lavender essential oil - 3 drops

Rose essential oil - 1or 2 drops

Usage:

1. Add these essential oils to 2 ounces of distilled water in a spray bottle.

2. Spray often in your work area.

Overcoming Insecurity

Essential oils can help to enhance self confidence and strengthen your emotions when you are feeling insecure.

Bergamot essential oil - 2 drops

Cedarwood essential oil - 2 drops

Frankincense essential oil - 1 drop

Usage:

1. Multiply this recipe by 4 to make 20 drops. Keep in a dark glass bottle then use the necessary number of drops in a diffuser.

2. For bath oil, multiply this recipe by 3 to make 15 drops then mix with 2 ounces of Jojoba oil in a dark glass bottle. Use 1-2 teaspoonfuls per bath.

Loneliness Diffuser Blend

This blend is helpful when you feel lonely.

Bergamot essential oil - 8 drops

Frankincense essential oil - 8 drops

Rose essential oil - 4 drops

Usage:

1. Mix together properly in a dark bottle.

2. Use appropriate drops in a diffuser.

Loneliness Bath Oil

Bergamot essential oil - 6 drops

Frankincense essential oil - 6 drops

Rose essential oil - 3 drop

Jojoba oil - 2 ounces

Usage:

1. Blend oils together in a dark glass bottle.

2. Use 1-2 teaspoonfuls in your bath water.

Panic And Panic Attacks Diffuser Blend

Use this blend in times of panic.

Lavender essential oil - 16 drops

Rose essential oil - 4 drops

Usage:

1. Add oils to a dark glass bottle and shake together.

2. Use this blend in your diffuser.

Panic And Panic Attacks Bath Oil

Lavender essential oil - 12 drops

Rose essential oil - 3 drops

Jojoba oil - 2 ounces

Usage:

1. Mix essential oils with Jojoba in a dark glass bottle.

2. Add 1-2 teaspoons to your bath water.

Emotional Shock Relief

Emotional shock can occur when you hear bad news or experience a negative occurrence. The following essential oils can help you to calm down until normalcy returns.

Lavender

Neroli

Tea Tree

Rose

Roman Chamomile

Usage:

1. Keep a vial of any of these oils in a purse or pocket.

2. Place a few drops on tissue or cotton ball and inhale. You could also use a nasal inhaler.

3. Mix any of the oils with a little carrier oil for a back rub or foot rub.

ESSENTIAL OIL RECIPES FOR WOMEN ISSUES

Vaginitis (Virginal Inflammation)

This condition is mostly caused by a bacteria and very rarely fungal infection. 75% of women will experience this condition in their lifetime.

Lavender and Melaleuca- 2 - 5 drops each

Extra Virgin Coconut Oil- 1 tablespoon (1/2 ounce)

Usage:

Add essential oils to coconut oil. Soak into a tampon. Use nightly for a week

Mood Soother For PMS

PMS is the acronym for premenstrual syndrome. It comprises various symptoms that generally begin several days before menstruation. These symptoms include breast swelling and tenderness, water retention, depression, irritability, headaches and mood swings.
Geranium essential oil - 9 drops

Chamomile essential oil - 6 drops

Clary sage essential oil - 3 drops

Angelica essential oil (if available) - 3 drops

Marjoram essential oil - 2 drops

Vegetable essential oil - 2 ounces

Usage:

1. Combine all ingredients. The angelica oil works real well but it is optional because it may be hard to find.

2. Add 1- 2 teaspoons to bath or use as massage oil. For more effectiveness, add 1- 2 drops of Neroli, jasmine or rose. Without the vegetable oil, it can be used in a diffuser or place in a vial to smell as needed.

Bloating & Headache Relief Blend

Lavender essential oil - 6 drops

Juniper berry essential oil - 3 drops

Birch essential oil - 2 drops

Patchouli essential oil (optional) - 1 drop

Usage:

1. Combine ingredients. Add 1- 2 teaspoons to bath1 teaspoon to a foot bath. It can also be used as massage oil or add 1 to 2 teaspoons to your bath. Patchouli is optional on account of its overwhelming smell so do not use if you cannot stand it.

Varicose Veins Essential Oil Blend

Veins in the body may become weakened with time and lots of pressure. As a result, they become enlarged and twisted.

Cypress essential oil - 30 drops,

Lavender - 20 drops

Lemon essential oil- 10 drops

Coconut oil - 2 oz

Usage:

1. Blend all and apply morning and night. Improvement will be noticeable in about a month.

2. When this happens, apply daily for 3 or 4 months more.

Essential Oil Preparation For Painful Periods/Cramps

Clary Sage/Cypress: 2-4 drops

Usage:

Apply topically to the abdomen. Next, use a warm compress on the abdomen.

Candida Or Yeast Infection

Lemon essential oil - 5 drops

Melaleuca essential oil - 5 drops

Oregano essential oil - 3 drops

Usage:

1. Add the essential oils to a gel cap then take internally two times daily for about 10 to 14 days.

2. Take a two weeks break then repeat the procedure.

Vaginal Candida Or Yeast Infection Douche

Geranium essential oil - 1 drops

Tea Tree essential oil - 2 drops

Rosemary essential oil - 2 drops

Lavender essential oil - 2 drops

Vinegar - 2 tablespoons

Lukewarm water - 3 cups

Usage:

1. Mix ingredients together.

2. Use once daily as a douche or Sitz bath.